Demystifying Hospice

Demystifying Hospice

*Inside the Stories of
Patients and Caregivers*

Karen J. Clayton

ROWMAN & LITTLEFIELD
Lanham • Boulder • New York • London

This book is written as a source of information and encouragement. The information contained in this book will be helpful but should not be considered a substitute for the advice, decisions, or judgments of the reader's family members and financial, medical, or other professional advisors.

All efforts have been made to ensure the accuracy of the information contained as of the date published. The author and publisher disclaim responsibility for any adverse effects arising from the use or application of the information contained herein.

As I honor my patients, caregivers, family members, and colleagues, their names, locations, and identifying information have been changed to assure their privacy.

Published by Rowman & Littlefield
An imprint of The Rowman & Littlefield Publishing Group, Inc.
4501 Forbes Boulevard, Suite 200, Lanham, Maryland 20706
https://rowman.com

Unit A, Whitacre Mews, 26-34 Stannary Street, London SE11 4AB,
United Kingdom

British Library Cataloguing in Publication Information Available

Library of Congress Cataloging-in-Publication Data

Names: Clayton, Karen J., author.
Title: Demystifying hospice : inside the stories of patients and caregivers / Karen J. Clayton.
Description: Lanham : Rowman & Littlefield, [2018] | Includes bibliographical references and index.
Identifiers: LCCN 2018006775 (print) | LCCN 2018012121 (ebook) | ISBN 9781538114957 (Electronic) | ISBN 9781538114940 (cloth : alk. paper)
Subjects: LCSH: Hospice care. | Terminally ill--Care. | Terminally ill--Family relationships. | Caregivers.
Classification: LCC R726.8 (ebook) | LCC R726.8 .C548 2018 (print) | DDC 616.02/9--dc23
LC record available at https://lccn.loc.gov/2018006775

♾ ™ The paper used in this publication meets the minimum requirements of American National Standard for Information Sciences Permanence of Paper for Printed Library Materials, ANSI/NISO Z39.48-1992.

Printed in the United States of America

To Dale, who shared it all with patience and grace:
friendship, marriage, children, my social work career,
graduate studies, teaching, museum work, traveling,
and the adventure of writing this book.

And in memory of my mother, my father, and Nan.
Each treasured, each of them left us much too soon.

Contents

Acknowledgments

This book exists because of my hospice patients, caregivers, and families. I honor them and thank them for sharing their lives with me, teaching me about living and dying.

My hospice and hospital colleagues and American Cancer Society family modeled how to work as a team, make a positive difference in people's lives, and give hope. Thank you.

My husband, an excellent writer himself, my rock, supporter, editor, and encourager, who stayed positive, patient, and kind and loved me through it all. There will never be enough thanks.

Our Oak Harbor Writing Group: Kelly Gust, Patrick Craig, Bill Walker, Erika Jenkins, Dale Clayton, and Ina Orme—a creative group of folks excited about writing in many different genres, who read and read and reread, critiqued, and loved my book. Huge thanks.

Much appreciation to my acquisitions editor, Suzanne Staszak-Silva, challenging me with a new format that I learned to love, quizzing me, answering my questions, guiding me through putting it together. Thanks to assistant acquisitions editor, Mary Malley, for her kind and quick responses and good information.

Thanks to Chris Fischer at Rowman & Littlefield for skillfully guiding my book through the many steps of production with patience and kindness, and to Kim Giambattisto, my necessary detail person. I appreciate Kelly Quarrinton's counsel in the complex world of publicity and social media.

Thanks to the Rowman & Littlefield Publishing Group, my first choice because they make it possible for readers, educators, health care professionals, social workers, spiritual guides, administrators, librarians, and patients, caregivers, and family members to have easy access to this information.

Agent Nancy Rosenfeld of AAA Books Unlimited, thank you for being excited about my project, encouraging me, and working fast and well to acquire just the right publisher.

I honor and thank my teachers and mentors who helped me understand the world in a bigger way: Frank Knittle (RIP) who urged me to ignore the freshman comp syllabus and get on with writing some bigger things; Bob Gardner, who opened my mind to sociological thinking and helped me put my world together in a meaningful way; John Jones, who opened the world of belief systems that affect everything I do; Doug Clark, who prophetically saw and contributed to my bigger interests; Charles Teel (RIP), model for justice and social activism; Gottfried Oosterwal (RIP), who guided me in medical anthropology; and Eugene Ramsey, irreverent and always pushing me to do the new and innovative and to choose what I really want to do. Thanks especially to Terese Thonus, teacher, writer, and author and my friend, and model in so many ways.

Friends who give me joy, help me really see and understand myself, help me think and believe in myself, who know me well, and continue to see the good in me. They are vital to me, my view of myself, and my courage. Too many important ones to mention them all, but for sure I'll include huge thanks to Elaine and Karen, my almost sisters since grade school, Liz and Liz, Ellen, Jann, Renee, Beth, Valerie and Marilyn, Janet, Jan, Audrey, and Bonnie.

Family—my organized and thoughtful father, my tender and encouraging mother, my kids and grandkids who give me joy and hope for the future, my sister, Carol, and adopted brothers, Chris, Tim, and Robin—thanks to each of you for being there for me always.

Introduction

WHY HAVE I WRITTEN THIS BOOK?

Hospice is extraordinary! I write to share stories about my patients who chose hospice care and focused on quality of life instead of quantity of time. They were more comfortable physically and emotionally than they had thought possible as their caregivers and the hospice team worked together to make the end of their life the best it could be. It is my passion to help readers become more comfortable accepting or requesting hospice comfort care when no more treatment for cure is available or desired.

Caregiving at the end of life is one of the final expressions of love. When people are very ill, they usually want to be at home with those they love, symptoms controlled, sharing stories, playing games with children or grandchildren, and eating brownies. Throughout history and in most cultures, families have offered that care, and hospice makes it possible for them to do so again. I want to encourage the forty million caregivers in the United States, 40 percent of whom are men, and inform them how they can have help with this difficult and complicated work. Most of us will likely become a caregiver to a spouse, child, parent, sibling, or friend. These stories will lift your spirits, touch your heart, and teach about hospice care.

This is a gentle book about a difficult subject. Through these stories you will better understand the interdisciplinary hospice team. I honor them: physicians, nurses, chaplains, home health aides, therapists, and volunteers. You will learn about my role as hospice social worker, offering emotional support and practical help to patients, caregivers, and other family members, including children of all ages.

Every adult needs to understand care options at the end of life. Accidents and chronic and sudden illnesses bring difficult decision-making to people of all ages. The more you know about your choices, talk to your family and friends about end-of-life care, decide the kind of care you want and don't want, and follow through by creating your own advance directives, the more likely the end-of-life experiences will be easier and less stressful, and family members will walk more easily through their grief.[1] Sophia's story will help you learn how to comfortably talk with your family and with physicians about end-of-life choices.

Hospice personnel continue to care for family members after their loved one has died, visiting, phoning, and inviting them to bereavement support groups. I'm honoring death doulas, who sometimes assist families in their home in the last critical hours, and administrators of retirement centers, assisted living and skilled nursing facilities, board and care homes, and other facilities that welcome hospice teams to assist their own staff and make life easier for patients and families. Our hospice chaplain and I often helped the family plan and present a memorial, funeral, or graveside service. I honor funeral home directors and home funeral and green burial advocates.

One evening I was sharing memories and tears with two different families at two separate "viewings" in one of the funeral homes many of our families used. The funeral director and I had worked with each other many times. As I was leaving that evening, he said, "I don't know how you do this."

I laughed and responded, "Hasn't anyone ever said that to *you*?"

"Yes," he said, "But you really *know* these people."

Yes, I knew them, visiting many of my patients and their caregivers over several weeks, sometimes months. Each story in this book emphasizes the treasure each life is, no matter how long or short. You'll laugh about Sara's bucket list, be touched by the "his, hers, ours, and theirs" family, honor several delightful military men, and learn how hospice helped a mom be able to care for Julie, her daughter, when she was released from prison. People can do extraordinary things with the right help.

The word "hospice" comes from the same root word as "hospitality." In medieval times, hospices were places of rest and shelter for weary travelers. Dame Cicely Saunders began the first hospice, St. Christopher's, in London in 1948, and now these services are available in many countries around the world. The first hospice established in the United States was Connecticut Hospice in Branford, Connecticut, in 1974. That same year legislation was introduced into Congress for federal funding for hospice; it did not pass. The Joint Commission on Accreditation of Hospitals Funding initiated hospice accreditation in 1982 and the Medicare Hospice Benefit was made permanent by Congress in 1986.[2] My father and I cared for my mother during her ten-year cancer experience and her death in 1983. We did not have the blessings hospice offers. I'm sure that made my work even more important and precious to me.

I'm sharing these stories of my patients, their caregivers and other family members, and my team, which have followed me in every aspect of my life so others will learn the blessings of hospice. Being part of a hospice, sharing the lives and deaths of my patients, experiencing the bravery and caring shown between them and their families and our hospice team all provide an excellent model of life-affirming love. Some names and locations have been changed to assure privacy.

WHAT IS HOSPICE AND HOW DOES IT WORK?

- **Hospice is "considered to be the model for quality, compassionate care for people facing a life-limiting illness or injury.** Hospice care involves a team-oriented approach providing medical care, symptom management, emotional and spiritual support expressly tailored to the patient's needs and wishes. Support is provided to the patient's loved ones as well. At the center of hospice and palliative care is the belief that each of us has the right to die pain-free with dignity, and that our families will receive the necessary support to allow us to do so."[3]
- **End-of-life specialists visit regularly** and provide needed assessment, coordinated medical care, medical equipment, medications, social work, and spiritual support. An assessment is made at three-month intervals, validating that the patient remains eligible. Patients who improve can be discharged until hospice is needed again. They can revoke the care at any time.
- **Six months of hospice care** are a benefit of Medicare, Medicaid, VA Benefits, and many other insurance programs; usually, there is usually no cost to the patients or their family. Approximately 80 percent of hospice care is paid by the Medicare Hospice Benefit (MHB).[4] A few private hospices operate without taking federal monies.[5]
- **Care is provided where the patient lives**—in his or her own home, with a family member, in a retirement center, a board and care home, or a skilled nursing facility. Hospice care helps avoid the often debilitating cycles of visits to physicians' offices, the ER, the ICU, or hospital stays. Hospice care is the most efficient way to use Medicare and other insurance monies, costing less than more aggressive treatment. Some hospices have a hospice house or a room or unit in a medical facility that can be used when care goes beyond the family's abilities.[6] There are many unique hospice arrangements.[7]
- **Palliative care is specialized care for patients with serious illness.** The goal is to provide relief from symptoms, pain, and the physical and mental stresses, and to increase the quality of life of the patient and their caregivers. Palliative care continues as the patient moves into hospice care when a

patient is considered to have six months to live. "People coping with serious illness who are under palliative care have better quality of life and suffer fewer symptoms than those who don't receive palliative care."[8]

• **Hospice care is available when:**

    a. A physician refers his or her patient to hospice when he or she believes the patient has a likelihood of not living more than six months.

    b. A patient or his or her caregiver[9] requests a hospice representative visit them; a nurse and often the social worker assess the patient and describe the services to the patient and his or her caregiver and other family members. If the patient is appropriate for hospice (there is no more curative treatment available or the patient doesn't desire more treatment), the nurse contacts the patient's physician who, if he or she agrees with the hospice assessment, signs the papers that qualify the patient for care. The hospice medical director also signs the agreement.

In 2016, 4,382 Medicare-certified hospices operated in the United States; 1.43 million Medicare beneficiaries were enrolled for at least one day. The average length of stay was seventy-one days. For-profit tax status hospices accounted for 62.5 percent of active Medicare providers and 24.7 percent accounted for not-for-profit tax status; 12.8 percent were government-owned providers. Including Medicaid, VA, and other insurances, the total is estimated to be 1.6 to 1.7 million.

It's difficult for any of us to imagine the world without our loved ones or ourselves in it. We grieve from diagnosis to death and after. Hospice personnel help at every step along the way.

It's stunning that in 2016 about one-third of hospice patients waited until the last week of their lives to use hospice care, and 40 percent had this extraordinary care for two weeks or fewer.[10] Chapter 10 identifies some of the mixed feelings about hospice that keep patients, caregivers, other family members, and health care professionals from being comfortable choosing hospice sooner.

My passion is to help you be comfortable asking for hospice help and, when possible, receiving the full six months of care that is offered. These stories will show you what a blessing hospice care is to the patient, caregiver, and other family members, including small children. My life is richer and my memories are precious because I've known these extraordinary people.

Chapter One

First Visits by the Social Worker

Hospice patient care begins when the assessment nurse visits, the patient's physician or nurse practitioner agrees to hospice care, and the appropriate papers are signed. A nurse is assigned to the patient and visits regularly, often twice a week. The social worker sometimes goes with the nurse on that first visit; otherwise, he or she sees the patient within the first five days. After the initial assessment, I saw my patients about every two weeks, and other times as needed. [1]

My first visit was carefully planned, and my goal was to meet with my patient and his or her caregiver together. On other visits I'd meet with the patient or the caregiver or other family members, often including grandchildren. Some of the meetings were away from the patient, occasionally at a restaurant, so the caregiver could talk privately with me, giving him or her a break from the moment-by-momentness of caregiving. A friend, family member, or hospice volunteer stayed with the patient during that time, having their own private time together.

I provided information about community resources, discussed patient care and grief, talked about their support system, invited them to community support groups, guided them in receiving financial help when that was appropriate, and assisted if there needed to be a change in housing arrangements.

Our chaplain and social workers created a kids' group, taking young grandchildren and children to ball games, to play miniature golf, or out for pizza, always finding time to talk about their family and their fears and providing opportunities to share their experiences with other kids.

Our weekly staff meetings and the patient file, including medical and social history, informed me of changes in patient needs, described family members needing extra attention, and even let us all know if there was an aggressive dog to watch out for!

My first visit was so important. My goals for that particular visit were to get acquainted, listen to any part of his or her story the patient wanted to share, offer emotional support, let him or her know the team was available 24/7, learn about the family and others in his or her support system, and give him or her an idea of the many kinds of practical, personal help I could offer. I usually discussed grief a bit—current grief and anticipated grief—and reminded him or her of the chaplain's help. You'll see when we meet Jenny and Mac and get past the story of the three-legged pig.

MAC AND THE THREE-LEGGED PIG

"This is likely the most difficult thing that's ever happened to you two . . ."

Our hospice nurses warned me about Mac, saying: "He's as irreverent as they come." They told me of his jokes, not unkind, but pointed, and one in particular. For example, our hospice was part of the Seventh-day Adventist (SDA) health care system. SDAs don't eat pork. Mac assumed each person on the hospice team was an Adventist, and he told everyone the story about the pig.

> A while back, I was ridin' my bicycle down a country road 'roun here, an' I saw this guy walkin' toward me with a pig on a leash. That was odd enough, but when I got closer I saw the pig had one wooden leg. Well, I had to ask 'im about that, and the farmer said: "This here pig's a mighty special pig. You see that house up there on the hill? That's my house, 'n a few days ago this pig woke me up in the middle o' the night, squealin'. He squealed so much I got up to try 'n shut 'im up, and I smelt smoke. Our house was on fire!!!"
>
> I told 'im that *was* mighty impressive, 'n I asked him, But what does that have to do with this pig havin' a wooden leg 'n bein' on a leash? And he said, "You see that well over there? Well, my young'n come up missin' one day 'n this pig grabbt holt o' my pant leg 'n got me t' go over there, 'n there was my young'n down in the well. If that pig hadn't got me t' go over t' that well, my young'n mighta gone 'n drowned."
>
> I told 'im that yes, that pig did seem mighty special. But still, why did he have a wooden leg? And the farmer said t' me, "Well, mister, ya don't eat a pig like that all in one meal."

Mac laughed the hardest of anyone every time he told that story, and he told it to anyone he thought even *might* be an SDA. Our chaplain, Marty, told me that Mac reminded him of that story every time they talked. Mac loved to talk and tease—he loved humor. He did *not* like to talk about his cancer diagnosis or prognosis. His energy was limited, but his symptoms were well managed, and it was likely he would live at least another three or four months after admission.

Jenny, Mac's wife, greeted me at their front door the first time I visited. She was upbeat and friendly, a delight really—strong, classy, and almost tough. She said she was so grateful for hospice and appreciated everyone who came to help in any way. That first day she and I talked a few minutes in the living room, and then she invited me into their kitchen.

When she introduced Mac to me, he mumbled a sort of greeting, letting us both know he'd really rather be working on a small engine that he had spread out on newspapers on the kitchen table. He focused on the gears and tools, not looking up at all. *This is not what I expected*, I thought. *Maybe he's just having a bad day.* The smell of motor oil permeated the area. The familiar and welcoming smell of coffee brewing and what looked like homemade cookies over on the counter added to the aromas in that cozy kitchen.

"You're busy," I said. "No problem, we'll sit here at the table and you keep working."

Jenny and I sat across the table from him and chatted; Mac worked on the engine. I did ask him to tell me about the engine, and he gave a very brief description. "Lawnmower." Jenny brought each of us coffee, set a plate of cookies on the table, and they listened patiently to my typical first visit presentation:

"I'm sorry this is happening to you. It's hard to be so ill."

They were both quiet. "I'm glad our hospice team can help. I know the nurses are coming regularly and the chaplain has been here. You know you can call any of us anytime. A special thing about hospice is that you're not dealing with this by yourselves anymore, you're not alone." Nods from Jenny. Nothing from Mac. Next, I asked them about their support system: "Who's helping you? Do you have family or friends nearby or a spiritual community?"

"Mostly it's just the two of us," Jenny said. She described their extended family far away and said they didn't have a church community and didn't know their neighbors well enough to call them friends. "There are some friends in Dallas we used to camp with . . ."

Mac worked on the lawnmower engine, and the small sounds of his work created a background to our talk. Occasionally he looked at me, sometimes offering a really short comment to something Jenny said. Now and then he asked her to go out to the garage for a part or a tool. I said, "I'm here to offer practical help and to talk about your feelings about managing a serious illness. It can be exhausting . . ." And I told them about community support groups.

Then I said, "This is likely the most difficult thing that's ever happened to you two . . ."

"Oh, no," Jennie said immediately

Really? I thought. Her reaction had been quick and strong.

"No, the most difficult thing was the death of our only son eight years ago; he was fifteen."

"Oh, I'm so sorry; how terrible!" I said. "How did that happen?"

"He was in a motorcycle accident," Jenny explained. Mac kept working on that engine. "The police came to our door, told us they'd take us to Parkland in Dallas—you know, where President Kennedy was treated. They said we had to get there fast, that he might not live 'til we got there—that he'd been in a terrible accident and was badly burned. They said he'd had his helmet on, that the helmet kept him from dying at the scene."

"How awful. I'm so sorry . . ." And trying to find something positive in that horrific event, *silly me*, I went on: "But it is good he had his helmet on."

Silence. Mac focused on the engine. *Wrong again.*

Then Jenny spoke for both of them: "No, it wasn't good. If he'd died at the scene of the accident, it wouldn't have taken him nine days to die. We watched him die for nine days."

What can one possibly say at a time like that? My first and second attempts hadn't really helped. I felt at a total and complete loss for words, but not Mac. He turned a flat expression to Jenny and said, "Yep. And it ruined our marriage."

It was very, very quiet in that kitchen. The only sound was the ticking of the clock on the kitchen wall. Then, suddenly, they laughed. They laughed hard. I didn't know how to respond. The story was profound and the reaction was revealing. I realized that their son's death *was* the most difficult thing they had ever experienced together, but it certainly hadn't ruined their marriage. They obviously had a wonderful connection; they were happy with each other and happy to be together, and they were showing me they believed they could manage anything.

The tension eased and Mac joined our conversation. They both talked about hating to face this current crisis and Mac's increasing limitations—his loss of appetite and energy—and the expectation that he would die from this illness.

They had already learned one of the secrets of dealing with tragedy: remember your strengths. We talked about those strengths and how they were helping now. He even made jokes about the illness. They both benefited from Mac's humor. What a pair! We talked about how the humor they both enjoyed could help them now. That's when Mac told me the pig story.

For the next few weeks, I visited them regularly. Sometimes I talked alone with Jenny and other times she would go out to do errands or have coffee with a friend and Mac and I would talk. The nurses told me that Jenny was always there when they visited so she could make her report to them, hear their assessment and suggestions, and learn what she needed to do to help Mac. They never asked for a home health aide; Jenny did whatever needed doing. They were together in their home almost continuously—sometimes in the same room, and often they each worked on their own projects in different parts of the house.

On their thirtieth wedding anniversary, I visited them. I congratulated them on their marriage, their anniversary, and their strengths. Jenny left to do some shopping, and Mac and I talked for a while. Then I said, "Guess you'll not be going out to get an anniversary card, huh?"

"Cute," he said.

I quit being "cute" and said, "One reason I came today is 'cause I thought you might like me to go buy an anniversary card for you to give to Jenny. Would that help?"

He loved the idea and hated the helpless feeling of not being able to do such a simple thing. I asked him, "Do you want a funny one?"

"Not a funny one," he said.

When Jenny came back, I said my goodbyes and went to a nearby card shop, taking my time and finding just the right one. When I returned to their home, Jenny was surprised to see me again so soon. I just said, "I need a moment with your husband," and she grinned and went into the sewing room. I went back into the room where Mac was reading and gave him the card. Mac cried. I cried. What a privilege to do such a simple meaningful thing for them.

Mac and Jenny were in our care for several months, and he died peacefully at home. At Mac's memorial service, our young chaplain stood at the door of the tiny chapel, greeting a few of Mac and Jenny's friends, their hospice nurses, and me. We'd all been touched by both Mac and Jenny—her upbeat strength and his humor. Soon Marty and one of Mac's friends walked to the front of the chapel, and the organist stopped playing. The eulogy was read, there was a special song, and then Marty walked to the pulpit. He stood there quietly for a while—almost thirty seconds—taking his time, looking out at the folk gathered there, acknowledging our grief. It started to get uncomfortable. Then he began. His first words were: "A while back I was riding my bicycle down a country road 'round here, and I saw this guy walkin' toward me with a pig on a leash . . ." And then he hesitated . . .

It was really quiet for a few seconds. Tears were rolling down my cheeks, but I had a smile on my face. Then there were a few quiet giggles, a little laughter—then a lot of laughter along with "good memory tears." It seemed that everyone there remembered laughing at the pig story and Mac's other jokes. They remembered his wonderful personality, his dry humor, and his stories. The chaplain shared memories of Mac and offered spiritual comfort to Jenny and all of us. He asked if folks in the chapel wanted to share memories, and several did, telling their personal stories about Mac and Jenny. That service and those positive memories were a good start for Jenny's living with and managing her grief, all eased because it would be mixed with so many good memories—and good humor.

The hospice nurses, the chaplain, and I all visited Jenny in the following days, and we invited her to a grief recovery program. She had steeled herself for this time and she managed, blessed by her good memories of their life together and how she had helped Mac be able to die at home as he wished to do. No matter who it was who visited her, Jenny brought up the story of the three-legged pig. It was a touchstone between all of us—and an anchor for Jenny and her memories.

GERRY AND GLEN

"Why is the social worker coming? What have I done wrong?"

Gerry, our patient's wife, answered the phone when I called to make an appointment for my first visit. She said I could come that same day, and a few minutes later she welcomed me warmly. During that first visit, my time was spent entirely with Gerry. Our patient, Glen, was in the end stage of lung cancer, which had metastasized to his brain and was affecting his thinking, awareness, understanding, and communicating. He was in a hospital bed in their bedroom, sleeping most of the time now.

Our visit went really well, and Gerry and I were comfortably getting acquainted, sitting and talking about some of the things I like to share on my first visit: "I'm sorry this is happening to you both. You're not alone with this difficult illness—the nurses will come at least twice each week and they are available for questions or emergencies 24/7, and I'll be visiting every couple of weeks—more often when you'd like. . . . This is likely one of the most difficult things that's ever happened to you."

Between each of my comments, I had asked questions, and Gerry told me pieces of their life together: describing their family, telling me about Glen's personality and how his illness changed him. She said it had been hard trying to know what to do as he became weaker.

"Who is helping you?" I asked gently. At this simple question, Gerry became rather agitated, clenching her hands into fists, pumping them up and down on her knees.

"I need some help right now," she said emphatically. "Right this minute!"

"How can I help, right now?" I asked.

"So many things are happening all at once. You folks are giving us so much—new medicines, the oxygen, equipment . . . people coming and going. We already had a hospital bed—he's in it. Today they're delivering some other stuff: one of those bedside potty chair things, a wheelchair, a walker with wheels, a transfer stool instead of the shower stool—and I don't even know what else. Where will I put it all?"

It was clear that right now the extra equipment coming was her biggest stressor; at that moment, even that help seemed like too much all at once. Sometimes it just takes "one more thing," even if it's a good thing, to feel overwhelmed.

"His bed's in the bedroom," Gerry said. "I want it out *here* 'cause I think he won't feel so isolated if he's in the living room. And it will be easier for folks to visit him, and I can see how he's doing while I'm cooking, or on the phone, or watching TV. How can I get the bed in here? Where would I put it?" She couldn't imagine how to arrange things so everything he and she needed would be *where* it was needed.

"You've got just the right person right here at just the right time," I said quickly. "I love to arrange and rearrange furniture. It's been a joke in my family for years."

And so we began. Such a simple thing, but at that moment it seemed the biggest thing on her very full plate: how to fit the helpful stuff into her already full house. Soon we'd figured out the best place in the living room for the bed; the medical equipment company folk could move that first when they arrived in a few minutes. While we waited for them, Gerry and I moved the chairs, end tables, and the sofa to accommodate where the bed would be. We took a leaf out of the dining room table and moved it against a wall so it took up less space. There were places chosen in the living room, bathroom, or bedroom for the other "stuff" coming. We had it done in a short time. She was relieved and delighted—feeling more on top of things for that moment. While we waited for the rest of the equipment, we sat and talked.

Gerry said, "You know I do everything I need to do—shop, cook, clean, even bathe him—and I'm glad to do it. I know he won't live long, and I want him here with me in his own home. I watched him get weaker and talk less. It's very hard and it's scary. I really feel afraid sometimes—I'm afraid for now and for later."

"Gerry, you're dealing with so much right now, with many kinds of grief. I've read a book by the author C. S. Lewis who kept a journal about his grief after his wife's death. Something he said has stuck with me:

> No one ever told me that grief felt so much like fear . . . other times it feels like being mildly drunk . . . there is a sort of invisible blanket between the world and me. [2]

"People experience all kinds of feelings, Gerry," I continued. "You are in an abnormal situation, and grief is a very reasonable reaction to that. There so many normal reactions to grief: there's shock and anger and panic—and fear. Sometimes there are physical reactions—headaches, a tight, aching stomach. There's sadness, of course, and sometimes there's guilt, hostility, even depression about the situation. People often feel an aimlessness. Facing the feelings, getting help from books, our team, your pastor, and maybe even other professionals can give you hope and affirmation that you are stronger than you realize. We can help you through it all. We are all here for you just as much as for Glen."

Rather timidly Gerry confided: "I'm so frustrated with our son right now. I don't know what to do. He lives very near, but he doesn't come much. He says he doesn't like to see his dad like this. . . . Well, I don't either! But I need him here, and I think his dad would know he was here, and I think it would help."

"That must be very hard," I said quietly. "We know how he feels, don't we? You know how hard it is for you to see Glen so ill. It may help to tell your son that you *do* understand and then tell him: 'I don't like to see him like this either, but your dad needs you, and I need you. You can talk to him; the nurses say he'll likely know it's you and it will help.' The chaplain or I can meet with your son if you'd like . . ."

Just before leaving, I went to the file I carried in the trunk of my car and brought in brochures about grief. We said our goodbyes for that day; she thanked me and said she'd like to talk again soon.

The next day Glen's hospice nurse told me that Gerry had called her right after I'd made the appointment the day before. Gerry had sounded very worried and asked: "Why is the social worker coming to see me? What have I done wrong?"

"The social worker visits every patient," the nurse had told her, "just to let you know how she may be able to help." Gerry had accepted that, but she was still anxious about my visit. It seemed that in her thinking, having a social worker visit meant there was something wrong and that there might even be an investigation. She had been genuinely frightened about my visiting—and also believed she couldn't tell me she didn't want me to come. She hated the whole idea of seeing a social worker.

Even though I know some clients may be fearful about that first visit, I look forward to it. It's my opportunity to get acquainted and let them know the positives about my being part of the team, begin my emotional support, and talk about some of the practical things I can do. The first visit is one of my most important visits. I learned on this first visit with Gerry that it will be good for me to remember the negative expectations some folks have about social workers.

STAN AND ROSE

An in-charge kind of guy.

Stan wanted all the action and the company he could get. He didn't want to be or to feel alone. I learned that on my first visit. I'd phoned ahead to make an appointment, telling Stan's wife I'd like to talk with both of them. They lived in a pleasant, older, two-story frame home surrounded by mature oaks. When I rang the doorbell, Rose called, "Come in."

Walking into the house I saw her in animated conversation with a friend. She was gathering her purse, sunglasses, and keys, and said: "Hi, you must be Karen." Then looking toward the open door of a sunny room off the dining room, she called out, "Stan, the social worker is here."

As she glided out the door front door with her friend, she said, "This is my girlfriend, Sally; we'll be back before you leave." She had a shopping list in her hand and she was in a hurry. "Bye . . ." and they were out the door and into her car and on their way. *Are you serious? That's a surprise—and a bit frustrating! A change of plans for me,* I thought. *My talk with her will have to wait for another time.*

A strong voice boomed out from the other room. "Hello there, I'm out here."

Following the sound of the voice, I walked through the dining room, entering what looked like a large enclosed porch, bright from the sunlight coming through the windows along three sides. Many of the windows were wide open and I could hear cars going by, kids yelling, and birds singing.

"Hi, Stan. I'm Karen, the hospice social worker. What a delightful bright room—so many windows. It's wonderful!"

"Yep," he said. "I love it out here. Used to be a covered porch; the people before us closed it in. I almost feel like I'm outside when I'm out here and the windows are open."

Stan was sitting in a big old comfortable-looking recliner—and it was on a platform, perhaps ten inches off the floor. *Hmmm, wonder what that's all about,* I thought.

"I can see out better this way, I like it up here like this," he said when he noticed me looking at his unusual throne.

He motioned for me to sit on a chair near him. The outside noises competed with some muted voices; looking around I saw that the TV was not on. *Where are those voices coming from?* Looking over the *TV Guide, Popular Science* magazines, *Readers Digests,* and stacks of books on the table next to Stan's chair, I saw a police scanner. So as a background to our getting acquainted, we had hints of what was happening in his little town.

"You're not going to miss a thing, are you?" I said, indicating the scanner.

"Nope! I've always liked being involved—staying busy. It's good to be where the action is. Guess it started when I went into the army. It was a busy time 'n I loved it. When I got discharged I joined the navy! I've traveled around the world, and now I watch the History Channel, the military channels, and different news shows. I like to know what's happening in the world."

"It sounds like you've led a fascinating life. My husband and I love to travel; what countries have you visited? I guess I should ask what ports?" He listed off the ports, including Subic Naval Air Station in the Philippines. I told him I'd been there too, during the three years my husband and kids and I lived and he taught in the Philippines.

How delightful, I thought, *he loves talking about his life—it's good for him and helps me know more about him; I hope he's as candid about his illness.*

He continued, "I'm used to knowing what's going on in our little town. I drove the EMT van for a while; when I couldn't do that anymore they'd let me direct traffic at accidents or fires or parades. Now, well, I listen and keep track of what's goin' on from here. Wish I could be out there doing somethin' worthwhile!"

"Good for you," I said. "It's obvious you've been good for your town. I'm sorry this illness is keeping you from being involved—it must be very hard for a guy used to being so active to be so limited. Still, you've found a way to stay in touch with your town. What a wonderfully healthy thing to do! How are you feeling right now?"

"I feel wonderful. Well, I can't get up and move around like I'd like to, but I feel really good. Finding out you have cancer is a real jolt! But ever since those hospice nurses got me the right medicine, I'm not hurtin'. I signed up about three weeks ago and I had such bad pain then. But they've got me feelin' really good. I think I'm getting better."

The man in the elevated recliner, listening to the police scanner, had been and still was very patriotic and community-minded, a real "man's man" and an in-control kind of guy. He loved remembering and talking about it all. Slowly he'd had to give up activities he liked. I got used to the intermittent chatter coming from the police scanner in the background. I knew it felt good to him to have it on, and he'd be one of the first ones in town to know when something important was happening. He didn't feel alone. He surely didn't seem as ill as I'd been expecting.

After about forty minutes of talking about his life, family, travels, illness, and hospice, he did seem to be slowing down a bit. I noticed he was perspiring and his speech was getting a little slower. He stopped now and then, swallowing often. He rested now and then without talking, then went on. Then he said, "I'm not feeling so good."

"Tell me what's happening, Stan," I said.

"Well, I've been doin' so good. I don't understand . . ."

"Tell me how you feel right now."

". . . just getting really tired; an' kinda short of breath . . ."

"Stan, do you have any pain at all right now?"

"Yes, a bit. . . . Damn, I've been doing so good."

"Stan, I'm glad you've been feeling better—but you are really very ill. I can see that something has happened in the last few minutes. Please tell me *anything* you can about how you feel . . ."

I didn't want to put words in his mouth; open-ended questions are the best, but right now I had to know specifics. I certainly didn't want him getting up out of that recliner, a feat in itself on its ten-inch platform, and I didn't know if he had a catheter in place!

"Stan, tell me what's happening now. Are you light-headed? And when did you have your meds?"

"I hurt—and feel a bit queasy. Medicine? Oh, I quit most of them in the last couple of days. I've been feelin' so good . . ."

"Stan, I'm getting you some water. And where do you keep your meds?"

He told me where they were and I headed across the room to a tray with an array of bottles and vials on it. Each container had the instructions for the patient, information a hospice nurse would need to know. My brain and body went into overdrive.

"Stan, just rest right now. Don't get up," I said, using my firm *This is important* voice. "I'm not a nurse—I'm calling your hospice nurse. She'll know what to tell you to take and when. I can tell you that you can't just stop any of these medications without talking to your nurse, no matter how good you feel. Exactly when did you last have your meds, and which ones?" I asked as I dialed the hospice operator.

He finally realized this could be serious and said it had been more than twelve hours since he'd taken any meds, except the ones for his nausea. Several of his meds were time release—giving relief over a twelve- or twenty-four-hour period. When ingested it takes a while for them to become effective, and when they are taken regularly, the symptom (for example, pain, nausea, vomiting, diarrhea, constipation) can be relieved and managed. He also had some medication for breakthrough pain that was fast acting.

One of the blessings of hospice is that the team is available twenty-four hours a day. That meant I could phone the operator, briefly explain our dilemma, tell her it was urgent, and she would contact Stan's nurse or the nurse on call. During those few minutes I waited for the nurse to call back, I lined up the meds, read the names and directions to Stan, and asked him to be as specific as possible about what he'd taken when. By then he was perspiring profusely. I got him more water and said we'd get him some relief right away. In addition to the time-release meds, there was one for immediate pain relief, but I would not do anything until I talked to the nurse.

His nurse phoned us in less than five minutes. She asked the right questions, I gave her my best answers, then handed the phone to Stan. She asked him questions, told him what to take, and then repeated the instructions to me. Stan took the meds as the nurse directed, and in a short time, he said he was feeling some relief. The nurse stayed on the phone with us until he began to feel better. She said she would make a home visit that same afternoon to be sure that everything was in order and would give Stan and his wife more instructions and explanations.

"Stan, I'm staying with you until your nurse gets here."

As a social worker, it's appropriate for me to talk to him about the importance of taking his medication—to urge him to follow directions and make reports to his nurse with any changes or questions and to not make *any* changes in when or how he took the meds without his nurse's guidance. These moments had been frightening for both of us, and it was a dangerous but effective way for him to learn the importance of communicating with his team.

When Stan's wife returned, I described what had happened and told her the nurse was on her way. Rose was rightly very concerned. While Stan rested in his chair, she and I went into the dining room. I asked her if she knew he'd stopped taking his meds.

"I didn't know he'd stopped—but he complained about taking so many. He usually doesn't take pills—just toughs it out, whatever it is. He's heard he might get addicted to the ones for pain. I'm not surprised he stopped some of them. I'm so glad you were here."

"Me too. It will be good to have a serious talk with his nurse; she'll be here soon. I'll stay 'til she gets here. Be sure Stan's a part of that discussion. He needs to know more about his meds and why he was feeling better, and he needs to tell the nurse any concerns he has about anything. He told me he thought having less pain meant he was getting better. The nurse can help you both understand and reassure him he'll not become addicted. Being dependent on medication for pain relief is different than addiction. I'll get you some info I have in the car about meds; also, there's good information at the American Cancer Society website. And Rose, I'm glad you had some time away. It's reasonable, even necessary for you to have some time for yourself. You have a lot of responsibility; how are *you* doing?"

Quietly she said, "It's so sad. He loves to be out doing things. He's always been so active. I'm trying to act like everything's normal, but it gets hard. He misses his friends and the community activities."

"Let's you and I have lunch one day soon and talk more. Perhaps he has a friend that could visit while we're out or when you need to go for groceries. If not, we can arrange for a hospice volunteer. It's not a good idea for him to be alone. He and his friend or the volunteer can play checkers or cards or watch a ball game—or the military channels. Do you folks have any family nearby?"

"I really don't want him to see how protective I feel, but I know he can't be alone now. No, we don't have any kids and no other family close. Thanks, but your volunteer won't be necessary. Stan has so many friends. I'll arrange for one of them or a neighbor to come now and then, especially when I need to be gone."

That experience was a wakeup call for both Stan and Rose, helping them learn important lessons. They had to recognize how sick he was, that his illness really was life limiting—terminal. The meds had been making him feel better—that's comfort care—but they were not curing his cancer. They both needed to be open to and trusting of the hospice personnel. Stan, the military guy, was used to following and giving directions, but these challenges were altogether different from anything he or Rose had ever experienced. It takes time to accommodate to being dependent. They did well, Rose and I had our talk, and Stan lived for several more weeks.

I think of Stan when I read this from Adlai E. Stevenson II: "Patriotism . . . is not short, frenzied outbursts of emotion, but the tranquil and steady dedication of a lifetime."[3]

SUE

"I'm so sorry this is happening to you."

Driving through the flat brown countryside occasionally softened by a few rolling hills, now greening as the new alfalfa was sprouting, I thought about our new profoundly ill patient, Sue, in the end stage of pancreatic cancer. Her hospice nurse was seeing her twice each week, and she'd told me Sue was very weak—and quite cheerful. It's such a sobering thing to make your way into the life of a person who is dying.

Sue lived in a rural neighborhood of large lots and small mobile homes. Parking beside her well-cared-for home, I walked up five steps onto a small, wooden porch. Always the fixer, I thought: *We may want to arrange for a ramp to help them get her wheelchair up and down; we'll have to extend the railing too. And there needs to be a safer rug, possibly nailed down. . .*

I tapped lightly on the frame of the screen door and a bright, cheery voice called: "Come in!"

Opening the unlocked door, I saw a tiny, frail-looking woman in jeans and a t-shirt, sitting up very straight, legs crossed lotus-style, on a hospital bed set against one wall of her narrow living room. She was smiling broadly, and I said, "Hi, Sue, I'm Karen, your hospice social worker. I phoned yesterday . . ."

"Come on in here—I can't get up, but you know about that! Come right over here and sit down; make yourself at home."

I'd read her chart and knew her age and some of her medical history, remembering: *We're the same age. That could be me in that bed. Oh my gosh!* Seeing her brought it home to me: *This is the first time I've had a patient my age: fifty-two. Too young to be so sick.* She seemed so tiny and so very vulnerable, and she was *so* thin! Sitting on the chair next to her bed, I took one of her hands in both of mine.

"Sue, I'm so pleased to meet you. We're the same age! And I'm sorry this is happening to you! It's hard to be so sick." I don't use the words "terminal" or the term "life-limiting illness" when talking to new patients. First, I'd need to learn what she knew about her illness and prognosis, and I didn't know yet what she was comfortable discussing. She likely had only a few weeks to live, and I needed to find out how much of that she understood.

"I'm so happy for everyone who comes by," she said. "I'm alone most of the time; it's wonderful knowing people will be coming. Sometimes when I'm by myself for very long I'm scared . . ."

"I'm sure it is scary, being so sick—and being alone a lot. Tell me about your family, your husband, do you have children?"

Many people have never talked to a social worker, and some think they don't want or need to pour out their fears, thoughts, and the intimate details of their lives to yet another person. And some folks are eager for a listening ear. My plan on this first visit was to get acquainted and help her understand my role—giving emotional support and finding out what practical ways I could help. I was thinking, *She's so open and friendly. What's going on with her family? Why is she alone so much?*

"Sad, but we don't have any children," she said. "And my family lives a long way away. My husband works days; he leaves early. When he comes home he fixes supper."

"I'd like to talk to him," I said.

"Oh, that's not possible," she said, shaking her head vigorously. "He said he'd never talk to you or anyone else about this. And he won't be here when he knows any of you is coming."

"Just tell him I'd like to talk to him—anytime. I could meet him on his lunch hour—just let him know."

She said she'd tell him. "That's nice, but it won't work, I'm sure 'a that."

"Who is helping you? Do friends or neighbors stop by?" I asked. "Do you have a church family?"

"Nobody—well, one neighbor stops by now and then, but we're not close. Me and my husband, we don't go to church—I believe in God, that's important to me—we just don't go to church. And I'm not close with my family."

"My goodness, of course you're feeling lonely. Well, you'll have lots of visitors now—Marty, the chaplain, your nurses, and I'm so glad we're sending a home health aide. How is that working out?"

"Oh, she's wonderful; she comes Monday, Wednesday, and Friday. The nurse usually comes Tuesday and Friday. The chaplain has visited; I love talking to him."

"Maybe your husband would talk . . ."

Sue stopped me: "No, he won't talk to Marty either. He's already said, and Marty phoned and tried."

"Alright. I understand. And I'm glad you're comfortable with everyone— you're not alone anymore. I'll be here every two weeks, more if you'd like. Tell me about your interests and hobbies and what you like to read."

"I don't have hobbies, but I do like magazines—and TV. I watch TV a lot."

I said, "I'll bring some magazines; what kind do you like? And would you like some books on tape?"

"I like those women's magazines, and I like *National Geographic*. My folks got that for us when I was a kid. Not books or even books on tape right now; I have trouble concentrating."

"Okay, I'll round up the magazines and bring them next time—or send them with one of the team members."

We talked briefly about medical equipment and medication. "You know all that is part of hospice, right? There are no costs to you."

"It's so wonderful!" was all she could say, with tears in her eyes.

"Sue, how are you feeling right now?"

"I'm okay," she said. That's the response most folks give to that question, especially to a social worker, so I continued . . .

"Sue, do you hurt or have any problems or discomfort at all right now?" When asked that way, often patients offered more information, and Sue said, "I feel so weak. I hardly have the strength to get out of bed."

"That's very reasonable. Cancer takes energy from your body and it's normal to feel weak and tired. Have you described this to your nurse? Be sure and tell her if you have any trouble eating or any nausea."

It's important that she feels comfortable telling me or the home health aide, especially the nurse, any of us, anything about how she feels and about what worries her. Normalizing fears is vital to help a patient not feel out of control. Information lessens fear and stress; less stress can actually lessen some symptoms. The aide and I would make notations or phone the nurse with concerns or changes.

"When we know what's happening to you, when things change, we adjust the care we give you. Please tell any of us about your worries and fears and any changes. Has the nurse talked to you about the 'sliding scale' we use? Really, we use it for any symptom—nausea, vomiting, not wanting to eat, constipation, pain, even depression or anxiety. Do you have any pain at all right now?"

"No, I guess I'm lucky. No pain. Just the weakness."

"People with cancer often think they'll have a lot of pain—and that's not true for everyone with cancer. Studies show that about two in three cancer patients experience pain; it's higher for some advanced cancers.[4] If you do have pain, the nurses can help you manage it—and we can help you with your other symptoms."

"The nurse asks me to tell her how bad it is. I'm still learning about that 'sliding scale' thing. We're going to talk about it more when she comes again."

"Good. The 'sliding scale' means you can tell us how you feel by thinking of 0 to 10, with '0' meaning no symptoms at all and '10' meaning the worst you can imagine. It's a way we can understand if you need more or less medication. We want you to be comfortable. Sometimes we use drawings of the face—smiley to sad—so you can tell us how you feel. The nurse will practice it with you."

"Thank you so much! It helps to be able to tell someone . . ."

"Sue, it's a pleasure to know you. We have lots to talk about and I'll come back soon. I'm going to leave some things for you to read—some of it about grief. There are many ways grief can affect us. Sometimes it feels like fear, sometimes it makes us really sad. We can talk more later about that. Remember, we're just a phone call away twenty-four hours a day for questions or emergencies. You'll get a call back right away, and someone will come here if you need us. Unless you have something you want to talk about now . . ."

"Nothing right now. Thanks so much. It's all so wonderful. This whole thing made me feel kinda out of control. Now, I feel safe for the first time in a long time—such a relief! I'm happy for you to come anytime—I'll be here. Leave the inside door open when you leave, the screen door keeps the flies out and lets the bird sounds in. I like that."

It was spring, and I enjoyed the spring flowers on the drive home. Almost always there are beautiful things to balance the difficult. I used my driving time to reflect on the visit. *Such a difficult time for Sue; what a courageous woman. Good that some of her time is filled with hospice people. Some of her fears are being relieved. I'm looking forward to my next visit.*

"Hi. Yes, please come in the morning," Sue said when I phoned for an appointment a couple of weeks later. "Sometimes I'm too tired in the afternoon."

Tuesday morning was warm and sunny and Sue's windows were open. I asked Sue if she got outside much. "Danny takes me for a drive now and then. We like to go to the lake; he fishes. I can't do that anymore, so I sit in a lawn chair and look at the magazines you sent and watch him fish. Sometimes we take a picnic; sometimes he has to fix it. I'm just so tired all the time."

"Sue, has Danny started talking to you about your illness, about his worries?"

"Oh, no, he doesn't want to talk about any of it. He never was much of a talker; says he just doesn't understand cancer—and he hates it. He'll do whatever helps in the house—shop, cook, clean. He just turns away and gets quieter when I say anything about hospice."

"That must be hard for you," I said. "You're so outgoing, friendly, warm. People say opposites attract. Is that kind of like you and Danny?"

"Yes, and it's hard. And I try to understand. His mother died not too long ago; it was hard on him. He sees his dad and tries to help him some."

"So he has many losses to deal with." Then I asked, "Do you have photo albums? Can we look at them together?"

Sue told me where to get the albums and we spent a long time looking at them, talking about her childhood and her marriage. She loved talking about her memories with Danny.

"How about looking at these pictures with Danny, talking about your good memories?"

"That's a good idea! I'd love that—Danny will do that, the photos anyway. He won't say much, but it will be good to do that, remembering the things we done together. Thanks."

Sue lived just a few short weeks after that talk. I was sad that I wasn't there when she died. Other members of the team were with her and Danny. The chaplain helped with the funeral service, and he did get to talk to Danny a bit. He had experienced several griefs in a short time and it was hard for him. We let him know we were there for him when it would help. But he was used to grieving alone.

Chapter Two

Hospice Care at Home

The majority of Americans report that they want to be at home with the people they love when they are seriously ill. Several of "my families" were three-generation households, created because of the patient's illness, reflecting what typical care was until a few years ago.

"The majority of hospice care is provided in the place the patient calls home."[1] In 2015, 46 percent of Medicare beneficiaries (1,381,182) received hospice care at home. Other patients received hospice through Medicaid, VA Benefits, their private insurance companies, or they were nonreimbursable patients covered by foundation and other hospice monies. Medicare calls this routine hospice care (RHC). Figures are not readily available for freestanding hospices.

Caregivers may be family members or friends; some families pay for additional services in their home from community agencies. Some communities offer assistance at home, which can supplement family care, and the cost may be based on the patient's income. The hospice social worker can help determine services in your community.

When caregivers work away from home, they can sometimes use adult day care facilities for patients who are ambulatory. Lunch is usually provided and costs vary by community and are sometimes based on the patient's ability to pay. Patients who are well enough can spend quality time in community senior centers.

If caregiving becomes too complicated for the caregiver or family, the patient may be able to move to a long-term care facility, hospice facility, or a hospice unit in a hospital; those facilities may also be used for a few days of respite for the caregiver.

ANNIE AND KEVIN

"Kevin, it's never going to feel okay."

Annie was thirty-six years old, married to Kevin, and they had three children under twelve. She and Kevin had recently moved to a small college town. Their plan was that they each would complete enough education to meet their personal goals and secure a bright future for themselves and their family. First, Kevin would work while Annie attended classes. Then after Annie finished her licensed vocational nurse (LVN) training and could work, Kevin would begin work on his degree.

Theirs was a busy family: the children, two boys and a girl, loved camping, playing board games, and going to the mall with their grandma. The boys were into sports and the girl excelled in her school's "Gifted and Talented" program. They each had lots of energy, many goals, and the intelligence to meet them.

Annie enjoyed her classes and made good grades. Toward the end of the two-year course, she began having severe headaches. The doctors ran many tests. Annie continued attending classes and was preparing for her final exams when they were given the bad news: she had a brain tumor, a malignant, frightening presence in that beautiful, bright, blonde head. She didn't stop her studies. She managed the headaches and took her exams, completing the course with good grades (first things first), and then she had surgery. It seemed to go well. Three weeks after the operation she took the exams for her LVN license and passed with flying colors! Annie was done with her courses and licensing requirements, but she could not go to work.

Her physical condition deteriorated rapidly, and soon she was homebound. When she entered our hospice program a few weeks after surgery, her left side was paralyzed. She was very pleasant, quiet, and aware, seeming to understand most of what was said to her, but she couldn't "name" things—door, table, dog, son, daughter, mother. During the surgery to remove the tumor, damage had been done to the language center of her brain, resulting in "anomic aphasia."[2] It didn't seem to affect her basic intelligence, but did make it difficult for her to recall names, nouns, and verbs—the words that are so basic to understanding one another.

She couldn't say her children's names or say "mom." When she wanted to talk about her children, she indicated each child by flattening the fingers of her right hand and showing their height and saying "this one" or "this one." She did the same to indicate her mother, except she placed her hand closer to her body. She could eat by herself but couldn't ask for a napkin or any other thing—a fork, bowl, soup, toast, or jam. Soon she couldn't dress herself. I tried to imagine what it must be like for her and recognized how I needed to adjust how I asked questions, asking in a way that did not require her to respond with a noun.

Kevin helped. Her mom helped. The kids helped. Annie kept trying to do the things she'd always done to take care of her family, cooking simple things, cleaning the house, helping the kids with their homework, and going shopping with her mom. She tried so hard but her limitations increased. It was discouraging for everyone. She was so sad and frustrated, and she also didn't feel well physically much of the time. She was fearful. Fear is not uncommon—fear of what was coming, of difficult symptoms, and of being a burden.

"I've got some ideas about how you can help your mom," I said to the kids one day. "I've brought some magazines, and we're going to make a scrapbook for her. You know it's hard for her to say some words. This is going to help her let you know what she needs or wants."

The children, eager to make life easier for their mom, worked well together. The plan was that Annie would be able to point to pictures to show them what exactly she wanted or needed. So each page they created focused on objects in different rooms. For example, they created a page titled "Bathroom" and glued in photos of a tub, shower, sink, toilet, shelves with towels and washcloths, toothbrushes, toothpaste, deodorant, lipstick—all things she couldn't "name." Annie was sitting at the kitchen table when they brought her the scrapbook. They were so excited and hopeful, explaining what they had done. They asked Annie to point to a picture of the thing she wanted right then—she found the bathroom page and pointed to a washcloth and the kids ran and got it for her. Such a joy! It worked really well. The kids loved it and some frustrations were relieved—and I reminded them that *they* had made things easier for their mom.

The chaplain and I took Annie's kids on outings with other children in our kids' group. We went to a Rangers baseball game at the huge stadium in Arlington, Texas, we played miniature golf, and we ate pizza and ice cream. We all had fun, and at each event, we made time to talk about the sad and tough things they were experiencing. The kids shared their frustrations sometimes; often they just played and had as normal an outing as possible under the circumstances. Sometimes we talked about how to say goodbye.

As Annie declined further she needed to use a wheelchair, and soon she couldn't operate it very well. She could still say "Hi!," "Yes," "No," "That's nice," and "Love you." She could say "I'm sorry" and often did when she couldn't say the right words for basic things. She could say, "Thank you!" and did, often. And she could and did cry.

When I talked privately with Kevin about how he was doing, he often guided the conversation to the kids. That was reasonable; after all, he was taking care of the kids, doing what Annie could not manage, working full time, and he had started taking classes.

"I've read about alternative and complementary treatments we could try." Kevin shared some of the concepts and asked the nurse about them. He was exhausted, emotionally and physically. Annie and her mom thought he stayed away too much. He was busy—studying in the library, doing errands, grocery shopping—when they felt he was needed at home. He was so frustrated and sad and needed time away too, so he often took longer doing these basic things. He told me: "I've read everything I can get my hands on about dealing with this; I've read the books by Dr. Elizabeth Kubler-Ross."[3]

I encouraged his exploring this excellent information from Kubler-Ross, a Swiss psychiatrist and pioneer in America about death and dying and grieving—especially teaching about shock, anger, denial, sadness, and acceptance. She made a huge difference in American care of the dying.

One early evening when I was leaving their home, I asked Kevin to follow me out to my car, wanting some time with him away from the rest of the family. "This is such a difficult time," I said to him. "How are you doing, Kevin? How are things with *you*?"

"She cries, she's so sad. I want to help."

"Kevin," I said. "When she cries, hold her."

"I do," he responded. "But she just keeps crying."

"Hold her and tell her it's okay to cry. It's really important to let her cry about it, and for you to accept her sadness. You could say something like: 'This is a terrible thing that's happening. It's an awful thing for you and for the kids and for me. I'm so sorry this is happening to you; I'm sorry it hurts so much. Cry as long as you want to. I'm here to hold you.'"

"But I have to help her . . ." He was hugging himself with both hands, unconsciously trying, it seemed, to protect himself against this terrible enemy that was changing their world right before his eyes. I stepped closer to him and put my hand on his tensed forearm, hoping to connect and comfort.

"I know I need to help her and the kids learn to accept this. It's so hard," he said quietly. "We've talked about it a lot. I wish I could get her to *accept* what's happening to her. We've told the kids; they know what's going on, that she's going to die. Of course, we pray for a miracle, but I don't think it's going to happen. She just keeps getting worse. It upsets the kids. I talk to her about it and she cries. I don't know what more to do."

Now I understand what is going on, I thought. *Kevin doesn't just want her to accept what is happening, he thinks when she comes to the stage called "acceptance" it will feel okay to her.*

"Kevin, it's never going to feel okay," I said slowly, waiting for this thought to settle in. "Annie *has* accepted the diagnosis and yes, she *does* know she's going to die. She has accepted it all. That's *why* she's crying. Think what it's like for her: She's never going to be able to work as a nurse. That's not okay. She's leaving your three wonderful children and you, and her mom and dad and sisters, and on and on to everything you can think of that is important to her. It is never going to be okay. It's not okay that she's going to die. It's not okay for that mind not to be able to express itself or for her to not work as a nurse. It's not okay that that mind will not exist sometime soon." And I thought, *Please listen and take this in so you can really help her.*

Kevin was very quiet—it seemed he was trying to process the huge difference between acceptance of what was happening and having it be alright. And I kept on, wanting to help him understand.

"It is possible to be very realistic about an illness and a prognosis, death, but it still doesn't feel okay. You can accept it; she can accept it . . . and it's still not okay. It's terrible. It's a loss that can't be balanced in any way whatsoever. Acceptance takes time."

I was surprised at my own depth of feeling. I'm not sure I'd ever expressed those concepts in that way before. I realized how much I felt it and meant it and how helpful it would be to my other families. And from then on it made it easier to understand and give "permission" to other caregivers and patients for the Dr. Doolittle's "Push Me Pull You"[4] feeling that facing death evokes. It is important to understand the difference between acceptance and feeling like it's okay, feeling good about it. There's a difference between accepting a situation and finding it acceptable.

Kevin was quiet for another moment, evaluating what I'd said, trying to make sense of it, balancing Annie's not being okay in her situation with his need for her to accept it. Then he said, "I never thought about it that way, that both things can be going on at the same time. I thought I needed to help her get to the place where she wouldn't be so sad about it all."

"I'm not sure that is possible," I said. "It doesn't have to be okay. She will likely not stop being sad, Kevin. I think it could be such a huge relief to Annie and to you when you can let her know you accept and understand her crying and her sadness and show that you share it."

He was still trying to take all this in. I continued: "Remember, Kubler-Ross urged people to have open and honest discussions through all the ways grief affects us—shock and anger, depression. She also urged keeping hope alive."

"Hope!?" Kevin's voice exploded. "Hope! How can we have any hope?" That seemed to be almost too much for him to take in. I described my understanding of hope in this way:

Hope Changes

- First, we hope we won't get sick.
- When no cure seems possible, then we hope we can manage difficult symptoms.

- We hope for peace within ourselves, with our family, friends, and spiritual experience.
- Then we hope for a "good death"—without fear, without pain, with peace, with the people we love beside us, ready to say goodbye.

"Kevin, this is how you can help Annie. Take your time, think about it, talk with Annie, her mom, and your kids about hope. You can all do this—you can do it well. And we'll help."

Kevin did become more supportive, allowing real feelings to be expressed—his children's, Annie's, her family's feelings, and yes, his own. They talked together about hope. And it was a terribly difficult time. Annie grew worse; there were even more limitations. She and her mom spent lots of quality time, just the two of them. And Annie spent part of every day in a comfortable chair in the room where the kids watched their TV programs and played games, taking in as much as she could while they said and did what kids normally do. Sometimes her mom or one of the children sat next to the chair, held hands with her, and quietly watched the activities together. They had those precious moments. A lot of photos were taken.

There often does come a time when it's helpful to say to a person who is near the end of their life, when death is inevitable, "It's okay to let go, to stop fighting. We will be okay. It's not going to feel right that you are not with us; we will miss you and be so terribly sad. And yet it's okay for you to let go." That is different than expecting that her life ending would feel alright, it just gives her permission to quit fighting when she is exhausted and actively dying.

Annie and her family relied on their Christian faith; it helped them find some peace, and she died a few weeks after Kevin and I had that pivotal conversation. It was so awfully sad for everyone. It definitely did not feel okay, but was somewhat balanced because they believed they would see Annie again, trusting that God was in control. I urged them to remember all the things they had each done for her to make her life more comfortable and joy filled. They had many good memories and photos of their times together, all helpful to each one of them.

Hospice workers encourage patients to look for strength in their spiritual beliefs. All cultures and belief systems offer insights and explanations about death. Many teach about what comes after death. Even when death becomes acceptable, when the quality of life is diminished, there is a terrible feeling of loss and it does not feel okay.

Terry Tempest Williams, in her book *Refuge: An Unnatural History of Family and Place*,[5] describes her mother's strong faith and also her being ready to let go: "All mother said today is how much she wants to sleep, to not think or feel, just to sleep. . . . And, now it feels good to give in. I am ready to go." There are times, in an emergency room, an ICU unit, or at home, when heroic measures diminish the quality of life. When we choose comfort care only, we acknowledge that it is okay to stop fighting death. But life is precious and death never feels okay in our hearts.

SADIE

Sadie's Bucket List.

"Yes, I know it's on your Bucket List,[6] but I can't take you there, Sadie."

"Ah, come on. There's not much fun in my life anymore. It's something I've wanted to do for a long time; it's something I want to do before I die."

"Not gonna happen, Sadie." I was adamant. "You'll have to go with someone else."

"Well, I'm not going to ask Jim or my daughter to take me," she said with a grin.

Sadie and Jim lived in a two-story, white frame, early 1900s farmhouse on a large lot at the edge of town. Huge old elms shaded them in the scorching Southwest summers. Set well back from the road, there was plenty of space and shade for Jim to park "Big Blue," his eighteen wheeler. Sadie was often alone there while he was on the road for days at a time. They were both in-your-face, delightful characters. Their daughter and grandkids lived a short drive away in town and came by often to help, cooking and baking with Sadie—and just wanting to be with her. She had a great spirit and was fun to be around.

Limited in her movements because of her weight, her wheelchair, and the tether to an oxygen machine running 24/7, Sadie was bored and wanted some excitement. An entire book could be written about the many traumatic things that happened to her and her family.

Our hospice team members enjoyed caring for Sadie. She was a delight! Some people have places to travel on their Bucket List—Sadie's choice was nearby, and we learned about it after spending an evening at her house watching the film *Thelma and Louise*. She hooted and hollered and we all enjoyed the film immensely. The closest thing to "doing a Thelma and Louise" in her mind was going to LaBare, a male dance/strip club about fifty miles away. She urged and we declined.

That situation was a prime example of cognitive dissonance for me—I wanted to help fulfill any reasonable wish my patients expressed; however, I don't like the exploitation of men any more than I like the exploitation of women. Yes, I know, men and women choose to dance and strip, or almost strip. Still, I don't think most of them would do that if someone paid them the same kind of money for some other kind of work. But that's *my* thinking and an ethical discussion for another time. Part of our decision was that the nurse and I both were quite sure our Christian-based hospice employer would eventually find out and definitely not approve. For many reasons, we chose not to take Sadie to LaBare. "Sorry, we just can't do that."

A few weeks after Sadie became part of our hospice program, I received a jarring message: "Jim's gone . . . heart attack. I can't believe it. What will I do without him? It's so unfair. Please come over . . ."

Of course, I went to her home, hugged her, grieved with her. Our team helped her and her family with some of the arrangements for Jim's funeral. One special feature was parking "Big Blue" by Jim's gravesite before and during the graveside service. A huge blanket of blue carnations was draped over his casket, his blue ten-gallon hat on top, and Jim was dressed in blue.

Soon after Jim's death, Sadie moved to her daughter's house in town. The grandkids loved having her living with them because no matter what was going on she would find some way to look on the bright side. Now that she lived with her grandkids, the team members had more good opportunities to talk with them and support them through her illness. Sara, her early teen granddaughter, was in our kids' group and I talked with her privately, too, about her grandpa's death and also about how sick Sadie was and what would soon happen to her.

I wasn't able to be with the family when Sadie was dying, but I drove to their house to be with Sara and the other grandkids as soon as I could get there. The whole family was almost overwhelmed with grieving, dealing with both deaths in such a short time. Sara had become so close to her grandmother, and she'd written her a poem. It was a private message—she didn't want to read it at the service. I said we'd make sure it was put in the casket with Sadie.

After the graveside service, friends and family were talking quietly on the lawn of the cemetery away from the funeral awning and the coffin. Sara came to me in tears. "Karen, I forgot to give you the poem. I wanted you to put it in there with her."

"No problem, m'dear," I said, hugging her. "Come with me."

We found the funeral director and I said, "Mr. Thompson, we have a very special request. Please open the coffin for us; Sara has a poem for her grand-ma."

"Of course," he said and walked us to the coffin. We three turned our backs on the rest of the mourners, keeping this as private as possible. Mr. Thompson lifted the lid of the coffin and Sara put the poem by her grandma's hand, patting that hand one more time. It was a precious moment, a good beginning of healing for Sara. I visited the family a few days later and was available whenever they needed. Sara continued to be part of our kids' group for a while and helped some of the other kids deal with their losses.

Funeral directors are really employees of families. I wish I'd known that when my mom died before I worked with hospice. During the service we sat in the family section, listening to the music, the eulogies from her many friends, and the words of encouragement from the pastor. At the end of the service, friends filed past her coffin and out into the parking lot, getting ready to go to the cemetery. Our family was still seated in the family room when the funeral director walked to the casket and closed the lid. My son Jeff asked me, "Mom, is that all? Is that it? Can't I go see her again?" And I just said, "I'm so sorry, Jeff." I wish I'd known I could have gone to the funeral director and made it possible for Jeff to have time at the casket, that there could have been more time for all of us, right then and there, before we left for the graveside service. Now I know even that would not have been too late.

JACKIE

"Alone is alright—with the right stuff!"

Jackie lived alone and liked it that way. However, when her emphysema progressed and became end-stage COPD (chronic obstructive pulmonary disease) and it was a struggle to breathe, she became frightened. Her physician felt it was no longer safe for her to be alone, especially at night. She was a financially independent woman, in her late fifties, on disability and managing—except for "extras" like medical equipment and medication. Then her doctor told her she had a likelihood of living only six months, and that was jarring; she was grateful he referred her to our hospice. We helped get her stabilized with appropriate meds and equipment, including the one special thing she needed: a CPAP (continuous positive airway pressure) machine to regulate her air flow at night when the problem was at its worse. One huge hurdle to living alone was solved.

Jackie loved the visits of the hospice personnel, and those visits were a real bright spot in the day for us. She offered tea, coffee, or cocoa, talked about what she or we wanted to talk about, and crocheted or knitted during most of the visits. Her hobby was creating delightful little outfits for tiny newborns and sweaters, mittens, scarves, and hot pads for family members, friends, school kids, and for us.

"I seem to make more than I have people for," she told me. "But I'll find someone who needs these things—at my church or some charity. Here—I made this hot pad for you . . ."

It sometimes happens that, when symptoms are under control with medications and equipment and stress is relieved, the health of a patient improves. Jackie still had emphysema and limitations, but she was no longer considered in the "end stage" of her disease. It was a big day when she was able to be discharged from hospice. What a joyful and surprising event! Still, it was a little frightening for her. To make sure she would feel more secure and be okay, I arranged for an emergency telephone response device that she'd wear 24/7, and she had her CPAP machine and her meds.

Jackie was home alone again and it was alright. We asked her to let neighbors know she'd been discharged from hospice and to ask them to stop by more often. The names of two neighbors were listed with the folks who managed the emergency device. When Jackie pressed the button, almost immediately a dispatcher spoke to her over the speaker provided, and she and they made decisions based on her answers:

1. "Jackie, it's the call center. Tell us what's happening." Jackie would describe her need.
2. "Do you want us to phone a neighbor?" Sometimes it was a simple thing a neighbor could do, and if not, the next question was:
3. "Do you need us to send an ambulance?"

And if there was no answer, the service called an ambulance. She was all set; we made sure everything was in order and said our goodbyes! Each of her team members phoned her at least once to be sure everything was going well.

The next Christmas I received a holiday card from her:

> ***Merry Christmas & Happy New Year***
> ***From Jackie, an ex-hospice patient.***
> *Please share this with the team.*
> *I'll bet you don't get many of these!!!*

GORDON AND GINNY

"I wish I didn't know what's coming."

"The first thing I noticed was my leg not working right," Gordon explained. He, Ginny, and I were in their comfortable living room, he in a sturdy recliner. "I was pumping gas at the station, got out of the car, took the nozzle from the pump, turned to put it into the tank, and I just couldn't make my leg do what I wanted it to do. I decided I was just really tired."

"I didn't notice it the next day or the next, but then more and more my legs just didn't work like they should. Then I had trouble picking things up with my hands, and I went to the doctor. He did a lot of tests and a few days later he asked me to have my wife come in so he could talk to both of us. He said: 'I'm sorry to tell you that you have ALS. That stands for amyotrophic lateral sclerosis—like what that baseball player Lou Gehrig had.'"

"It was frightening," Gordon's wife went on for him. "We'd heard about Lou Gehrig having some strange kind of disease, but neither of us knew anything about it. We asked the doctor what that meant. He told us about it, and now it's really frightening . . ."[7]

"Yes," Gordon said quietly, "I wish I didn't know what's coming . . ."

Gordon and Ginny now knew that ALS affects the nerve cells in the brain so that it can't initiate and control muscle movement. Gordon was frustrated when his speech became slurred. The usual progression is a gradual weakening of the muscles, then paralysis. The good news is that the person's mind stays sharp; of course, that means the bad news is he or she is acutely aware of all the changes. The disease may come on very slowly and death usually occurs in a few months or up to two years; the vast majority of deaths are due to respiratory failure.

"The doctor told you, I'm sure, that sometimes ALS goes slowly at first." I wanted to be encouraging and also help them deal honestly with what was coming. "It's different with each person. We'll help you both however we can. It is a frightening diagnosis; a terrible disease. I'm so sorry it's happening to you. You won't be alone. And I want you to know I'll spend time with Kyrstin and we'll involve her with other teenagers in our kids' group."

When Gordon and Ginny became a part of our hospice they'd known about ALS for some time. They had already experienced many reactions to the terrible news: at first when Gordon was feeling good, they denied the diagnosis for a time; when he experienced muscle spasms or shaking, they felt panic and deep sadness. There was anger and fear. And those feelings came and went with each change.

They were in their mid-forties; Gordon had to quit his job, and Ginny stopped working to care for him. Fortunately, in Texas at that time, there was a fast track to Social Security disability status. We helped them apply right away. These applications usually went through quite quickly—and once approved the payments and benefits began with the date of application. What a blessing! Now Congress has waived the typical two-year waiting period for terminally ill patients to begin receiving benefits of Medicare under the Terminal Illness Program (TERI).[8] Just paying for the medications and medical equipment would have been difficult or impossible for them without hospice. The nurse visits and later the personal care from our home health aide were vital for Gordon and Ginny. They could not have afforded that help.

The nurses did their best to help Gordon manage the decreasing abilities. We all listened to his frustrations and fears and I helped in some very practical ways: His fingers became contracted and it was almost impossible for him to pick up or hold a pen or pencil and write. I arranged for a computer for him and helped him learn to depress the keys by using the eraser end of a No. 2 pencil held in his curled fist. That worked for a while; then he quit trying. He might have held the pencil in his mouth as some cerebral palsy patients do, but he became too frustrated. "Why can't I make them work?"

"Let me tell you a story," I said. "Grace Hopper, according to a popular legend, was in the military in the mid-1940s. She was so good at math and electronics that she was assigned to a team developing computers and programs. One day a computer stopped working, and she turned it off, opened it, and discovered a dead moth in the circuits. She removed the moth, turned on the computer, and—it worked! When asked what was wrong, she said, 'There was a bug in the computer.' Thereafter, when the computer wasn't working properly, they joked, 'Oops, there's a bug in the computer.'"

"Gordon, something in your nervous system is destroying your nerve cells—acting like that bug. Not funny, I know, but maybe easier to understand what's happening."

Everyone was challenged to find practical ways to help. We talked about the grief of limitations and loss of control. The reality of what was coming was the worst. Each limitation was a reminder, and he was fearful.

Gordon became more limited, using a cane to walk. Then two canes, next a walker, and then a wheelchair. Each change seemed like a step downward, making him more dependent. Then he became bedfast; we brought a hospital bed into a room in the front of their house. He could see his front yard, the sidewalk, the street outside, the kids walking or biking past—and he saw into the living room. The TV in his room helped distract him from his situation, entertained him, and kept him in touch with the outside world. Ginny and Kyrstin ate their meals there and watched TV with him.

He struggled to remain positive. He'd do alright for a while, getting used to the latest limitation, then something else would happen. Then he got a cold; the breathing was so difficult because his chest muscles were atrophying. As his condition deteriorated, he sometimes felt panic. At times he cried and begged Ginny to call "911" so he could go to the hospital. We supplied him with oxygen as needed at home, and the hospice physician and nurse were doing their best. He could, of course, have chosen to go to the hospital emergency room where he would likely be intubated. There could be two important consequences: (1) he might become dependent and it would not be possible to extubate him and (2) because the ER visit and the intubation would be considered a heroic measure, he would have to sign off hospice. He was encouraged by all to do what he believed was best for him, to consider if he wanted to be on a ventilator ongoing. He didn't. He just periodically got understandably really scared.

He asked about what to expect; we gently told him the muscles would continue to weaken, and when his breathing got more difficult, he could go back on oxygen. That would help for a while, but at some point he would not be getting enough oxygen, the carbon dioxide would build, and he would likely slip into a coma and thankfully not be aware anymore.

Gordon's swallowing began to be affected; sometimes he had trouble clearing his throat and his speech was garbled. It all felt like a downhill slide, and it was. In our hospice meeting, we discussed his fears.

"He knows he's going to die. We've talked about it—he talks about it," I said. "He's afraid of what's coming next and how he'll handle it."

"He says he's ready in a spiritual sense," our chaplain said.

"He knows it's coming eventually," said another team member. "I don't understand why he doesn't just give in to it. Maybe it's time for that. Now he wants a feeding tube."

"He doesn't give into it because he doesn't want to die," I said. "He's already given in to so many limitations. He's actually calmer most of the time than I would have expected. People can often get along with much less ability than they ever imagined they could, but this has been going on so long. The one thing I think may help him be more comfortable and less frightened would be that abdominal feeding tube."

Artificial nutrition and hydration are a dilemma in hospice care; they are viewed as life-extending measures and, when a person cannot eat or drink, it can mean that his or her body is shutting down and cannot properly manage hydration or nutrition. When that is true, artificial aids may actually make a patient uncomfortable. Some hospices have an "open access" policy that allows some aggressive treatment if it is seen as a comfort measure. Guidelines are available from professional organizations to help make these decisions. [9]

The team member who spoke up was not an uncaring person; she just thought we'd tried everything reasonable and everything hospice protocol allowed. However, I decided to push the team on this one.

"Gordon is not on hospice because he has a problem with his swallowing mechanism; his death will happen when the ALS causes all the muscles to stop entirely. The limitations will progress and, as we know, usually the last muscles that will remain working will be his heart and his eyelids," I explained.

"He has accepted his inevitable death. Much of the time he's very brave. He still has some quality of life, and he and his family feel it's not okay to stop if this simple procedure can help for a while. This is for his comfort."

The team agreed, Gordon got his feeding tube, and some of his stressors were relieved. The quality of his life improved for a time and he had a few more weeks with his family. Then he quietly slipped into a coma and was no longer in distress. He died peacefully at home with Ginny and Kyrstin.

Chapter 2

JAMES AND MADGE

The wandering mind and body.

Madge had many good memories. She and James had raised a family together, and each had their own careers. They had visited thirty-eight states with their travel trailer, camped, fished, and learned about America. Now retired, she loved to bake, he loved to fish, and they enjoyed watching old movies together. She wanted to talk about things past and present. James, never a big talker, was diagnosed with Alzheimer's disease, the most common form of dementia, and didn't talk much about anything anymore. Slowly he was less involved with Madge and had fewer interests.

When his doctors said he was in the end stage, Madge and the family chose to ask for hospice care. The seven stages of Alzheimer's move from "normal outward behavior" to "very severe decline." At that end stage, eating, walking, and even sitting up can be affected, and it's important to remind patients to eat and drink enough. The brain does not give appropriate messages and basic behaviors are severely diminished. [10] And there can be personality changes, with some patients becoming very quiet and some agitated.

James seemed comfortable at home with Madge, calm most of the time. He'd sit and watch movies with her or with his adult children who visited as often as they could to be with their dad and to help their mom. "So many patients and caregivers deal with this illness (which becomes a family illness) it is thought it may become the 2nd leading cause of death in America." [11]

Physically James had few problems, and he enjoyed walking. He wandered the house, unlocking doors and walking outside whenever he could. For a while the walks were in their yard, then the neighborhood, then beyond the neighborhood. Sometimes he didn't find his way home and Madge or other family members would search for him. Soon the family decided it was necessary for them to install deadbolt locks high on all outside doors. It worked for a while, then James would stand on a chair and work at a lock until he got the door open, then go out and disappear.

Researchers report that about 60 percent of Alzheimer's patients attempt to leave home; the term "elope" is used by some, others use "wander." "Every year there are an estimated 125,000 reports of critical wanderers, [and] . . . if not found within 24 hours statistics indicated that they have only a 55% chance of survival. It's a real problem." [12]

James didn't remember to take his meds and sometimes became belligerent when Madge tried to help. The nurses let her know which pills she could crush and which capsules she could empty and put surreptitiously into applesauce or ice cream. Then he didn't want to bathe or be helped with other tasks. Hospice offered a home health aide, a man, and James let him help.

Madge let him wander inside the house, but soon James could not safely be left alone. Madge was exhausted, physically and emotionally, trying to stay aware of where he was and what he was doing and being thwarted when she tried to help. Their children, a neighbor, or our volunteer stayed with James at times so Madge could shop or meet a friend for coffee or a movie. And she was so lonely. She came to understand the reason for the titles of some popular books about Alzheimer's disease, such as *The 36-Hour Day*[13] and *The Long Goodbye*.[14] With Alzheimer's, the brain doesn't send the signals for some basic everyday tasks. And it just keeps getting worse.

The chaplain and I listened, encouraged, and made suggestions, acknowledging the ongoing grieving she was experiencing, a sort of "ambiguous loss."[15] James was present physically, but their history and memories seemed lost to him, therefore not shared with her. At the same time, James likely was experiencing his own kind of "hidden dementia grief" as he lost mental capacity and couldn't remember names or recognize people.[16]

We looked at photo albums, I encouraged her to talk about her good memories, and urged her to look at the albums with James and the children too. Sometimes a photo would trigger a memory that was meaningful to him. The memory did not last long; they had that moment. Those moments matter. Research has shown that "endorphins released during a pleasant experience have a salutary effect on a person with dementia even after the experience is forgotten."[17]

Many helpful tools are available for the family of Alzheimer's patients, including:

1. Medical alert systems with GPS tools, which worked very well for James and made the wandering less of a problem;
2. "Family Caregiver Alzheimer's Training" free online;[18]
3. The Alzheimer's Association website and printed material about caregiver stress and dementia; and
4. State personalized help to report missing persons (check by state).

One memorable day, Madge and I were sitting at the kitchen table, drinking coffee, discussing the birthday party she was planning for James. When she drank coffee at the table, she always included a cup for James, and he wandered in and out of the room. He came and sat with us at the table, holding his cup, drinking his coffee. I turned to him and said, "James, what's so special about August 13 anyway?" And he responded: "It's the birthday of a very special person."

We were delighted and made a big deal about the party. He smiled, then got up and walked away, through talking for the moment.

There are many exhausting things about living with an Alzheimer's patient: the constant watchfulness required, the repetition of requests, answers, and questions, the loneliness of not connecting, and the sadness of not being with the personality you love and remember. About 5.4 million Americans, one in nine of those over sixty-five,[19] were diagnosed with Alzheimer's disease in 2016, "the degenerative brain condition that is not content to kill its victims without first snuffing out their essence."[20]

We talked about energy or protein drinks, like Boost© or Ensure©, which can provide nutrition and calories. Some folk like drinking it just as it comes out of the can—cold is usually best. I shared some ideas about making it a treat:

1. Make a milkshake: whiz the energy drink with fruit or chocolate.
2. Make a hot or cold mocha drink: dissolve one teaspoon of instant coffee in hot water; stir it into the chocolate drink.
3. Mix in fruit, coffee, and/or chocolate and pour it into a freezer tray; when frozen it's a bit like sorbet. *Be sure to check with the patient's hospice nurse first.*

James lived several more months on our hospice program; his abilities continued to decline, and when he became bedfast we increased the visits of the home health aide for personal care. The family was a wonderful help to Marge. After his death, members of the team kept in touch with Marge for a time and invited her to our hospice program's "Life After Loss" program offered in our community by the American Cancer Society. Some of the groups were facilitated by our hospice team members.

Chapter Three

Caring for the Caregiver

Each of us will likely be a caregiver at some time for a child, parent, spouse, sibling, or friend. We may become intimately involved in their end-of-life decisions. It is a precious thing to help someone you love through the last months, days, and minutes of life. The stories you and they create become a meaningful part of your lives forever.

The attention of hospice physicians, nurses, and home health aides is focused mostly on patient care; they also teach, guide, and support caregivers. The chaplain offers spiritual and emotional support to the patient, family, and the team before, during, and after a death, often assisting with funeral or memorial services.

It was my joy to work with caregivers as much as with my patients, and when patients were comatose my focus was almost completely on the caregivers and other family members.

There are about 43.5 million unpaid family caregivers in the United States, and 45 percent of them are men.[1] My patient Jack was also the caregiver for his wife, diagnosed with Alzheimer's. Another patient's family seemed a social worker's dream: eight adult children, and I thought of each of them as potential caregivers. But even with family conferences I arranged, many of them stayed distant. Janine was happy to be her husband's caregiver; she gave and gave and gave, and I urged her to give others the blessing of helping her and created a way to make that easier.

Our hospice team was a well-balanced partnership caring for our patients, their caregivers, and each other. We all were aware of the sadness, fears, and chaos end-stage illness can cause. The primary caregiver was identified, and the secondary caregivers—sons, daughters, and siblings—with their abilities to care were often affected by practical things like jobs, finances, and distance. In the book *Let's Talk about Dying*, email conversations about many aspects of caregiving and dying, Steve Gordon says, "There we often are, turning our lives upside down to meet the needs of someone whose needs are many, and whose time might be short." And Irene Kacandes responds, "Many of us are secondary caregivers, taking over for a few hours, days or weeks when we can, doing supportive work like laundry cleaning, or cooking" and continuing to take care of our own families.[2]

Many helpful books and websites with guidelines and insights about caregiving are listed in the appendices. I especially recommend these two books: *Passages in Caregiving* by Gail Sheehy,[3] who shares the story of her seventeen-year journey caring for her husband (Sheehy was AARP's Ambassador of Caregiving in 2009) and Paula Span's book *When the Time Comes: Families with Aging Parents Share Their Struggles and Solutions.*[4] The Conversation Project co-founder and director Ellen Goodman describes the "cascading number of decisions" she had to make as a caregiver herself; this and more helpful information are found at their website.[5]

The U.S. Senate (S.1028) and the House of Representatives (H.R.3759) have passed a new bipartisan Family Caregiver Act, titled Recognize, Assist, Include, Support, and Engage (RAISE). It now returns to the Senate for "language approval and consolidation" according to a Policy Alert from the National Alliance for Caregiving. The bill would require the Secretary of Health and Human Services to "to develop, maintain, and update an integrated national strategy to recognise and support family caregivers." The sponsor is Senator Susan Collins (R-ME).[6]

Caring for my mother through her ten-year cancer experience and death and my father for a very short time after his final stroke, were such touching and amazing blessings. I'm pleased to share some of my hospice caregivers' stories so others can learn from their challenges and triumphs.

The National Alliance for Caregiving and Global Genes are partnering to bring attention to rare diseases and their impacts on family caregiving. They have identified seven hundred rare diseases, with cystic fibrosis leading the list at 9 percent of the total. One in four caregivers are millennials; one in ten are seventy-five or older. Family caregivers are identified as facing physical, emotional, financial, and social strains. All family caregivers will recognize those concerns. In the rare disease category, 62 percent of caregivers are caring for children under the age of eighteen. Many of the respondants in this study said they had to train health care professionals in the needs of their child.[7]

MR. THOMPSON'S DAUGHTER

"Who's helping you?"

Mr. Thompson spent several days in ICU after a major heart attack. His physical condition improved; however, his diagnosis was end-stage heart disease, and his physician referred him to our hospice. When I visited him in his hospital room he was pleasant, but his conversation was very limited. He was discouraged and had little energy.

"My wife's already passed, 'n I just want my kids to decide what's next for me. Thanks for coming, talk to them . . ."

That seemed promising—several of his children were either in his room or in the hallway. We found a small conference room in which to talk. This family seemed like a social worker's dream—eight adult children, each with spouses and children of their own. I expected they could and would work with each other to help their dad.

Reality soon set in: seven of the children and most of their spouses were employed full time, and five of them lived more than one day's drive away. One son told me that the most basic decision had been made: "Nancy will be the caregiver. She lives nearby, and they have a big house with plenty of room. She is the logical choice."

"Nancy doesn't work, she's a stay-at-home mom," said another son.

I bristled at the phrase "Nancy doesn't work."

"All moms are working moms," I said.

The siblings saw her as unemployed and perfect for the job. When I turned to Nancy, she said quietly, "We have four children and a pretty busy household; we live out in the country nearby—and our guest room would work, I guess."

The other adult children were so pleased and relieved to have that decision made. No kidding! They appreciated what hospice would give them, and with all that help they were confident Nancy could handle things just fine. Before they left to go back to their various homes, jobs, and responsibilities, I urged them to make plans together to visit their dad regularly.

"It's important you plan your visits so Nancy and her family can have periods of time for themselves. All caregivers need to have breaks now and then." They said they would make a real plan later.

Nancy and her family's country home was large and beautiful. When I visited soon after Mr. Thompson was discharged from the hospital, she and her husband had already decided that the best room for dad was on the second floor. It had an attached bathroom, a great view of the countryside, and they thought it would be good for him to be away from noisy family activities. I wondered if he really wanted that. It was hard to tell; he was weak and tired and didn't talk much. He did sleep a lot, so the quiet was a good thing most of the time.

We set up a remote monitor so he and Nancy could communicate when she was downstairs. The room was up a grand staircase that he couldn't navigate by himself, and he was alone in the bedroom most of the time. Nancy brought his meals to him on a tray. I urged her to stay and eat with him when she could. She said she often really didn't have the time, busy with some activity with or for the kids.

"Who's helping you?" I asked two weeks later on my next visit. None of her siblings from out of town had visited, and there were only occasional short visits from the nearby siblings. Another two weeks, the same thing. Soon it was obvious that Nancy was tired and not able to be as involved with her own kids and their activities as she wanted. I asked for another family conference, hoping to find some relief for Nancy and better awareness for the siblings.

Three of the nine children met with me—one of the three was Nancy. The siblings who lived nearby said they would pass on any important information to those not attending. When I asked how they thought things were going, they said they were very pleased; Nancy said it was going alright. I firmly reminded them all that it was time to create an actual written schedule for all the siblings to be more involved, making sure that Nancy and her family had time away regularly.

"We don't know how to take care of him, don't know about his medications," said one sibling. The other said, "I'd be really afraid of the responsibility."

"Yes, I understand," I said. "Nancy was and is concerned about the responsibility; she didn't know about those things either before he moved to her home. She can teach you like the hospice folks taught her—and we'll make a chart about which meds to give when, and how to do it. There's a medication chart that helps a lot. And you can call hospice any time, twenty-four hours a day, just like Nancy does." Was I pushy? Yes, and determined. Then I reminded the siblings: "Nancy needs a break; her family needs a break. It's really important to have some time away from caring for your dad so she can have the energy she needs to keep managing her heavy schedule. And her kids need time with their mom, at home and at school activities. She can't leave your dad alone, and he can't go out with them."

I tried to describe to them the weight of total responsibility Nancy had been feeling for days and now weeks. "Nancy needs a break so she can keep giving the care your dad needs." Again, I urged the siblings to help her regularly and to pass my message to their brothers and sisters. And we created a care plan:

Father Thompson's Family Care Plan

- Each sibling is asked to be at Nancy's home at least one full day one weekend every two months, taking total responsibility for the patient care, supported and guided by hospice.
- Those living in town are urged to take turns, providing care one evening a month for at least four hours with hospice on call.
- All siblings agree to share in the cost of anything hospice does not provide (for example, paid hourly caregivers in addition to hospice, as needed).
- The nearby siblings will encourage the other children to make weekend visits to see the patient and to assist Nancy and her family.

The reality was: (1) the other seven children almost never helped, (2) Nancy was not willing or able to insist that they did, (3) I couldn't *require* their help, and (4) she didn't. I had to accept their choices. This family wanted their dad to be cared for by a family member; however, they were not willing to care for their sister. It's important for caregivers to discover and develop their support system, including family, friends, neighbors, support groups, church/mosque/temple members, community agencies, and books.

We provided Nancy guidance, gave her children books about caring for their grandpa, and urged her to think of people who could give her "time out." The home health aide was there for two hours three times per week; Nancy could be away for that time period.

Hospice offers respite care with the patient in a facility for a few days under some circumstances. With the potential of help from several children not realized, it's hard for hospice to agree to the cost of respite care. That was a real dilemma. And it's sad that the other eight children missed the opportunities to be with their dad in his final weeks and days.

It was much harder on Nancy than it needed to be. She wanted to care for him; she did it well, and she, her husband, and her children have good memories despite the stresses involved. Mr. Thompson died several weeks later in Nancy's home. Mr. Thompson's other children were not there then and had not done their part.

"Sometimes life surprises us and we find ourselves in unexpected situations like a loved one receiving a difficult medical diagnosis, an unforeseen accident, or an aging loved one needing help. Someone needs care and someone else becomes the caregiver."[8]

Chapter 3

JANINE

"Here's how you can help."

Janine was the primary caregiver for her husband, Henry. They had lived, worked, raised their children, and gone to church in a rural town all of their forty-six years of married life. When I visited the first time, Henry was already semi-comatose; I sat beside his bed and talked to him a bit (you never know what patients perceive) and then spent most of my visit time with Janine. We had a good talk about their marriage, their family, their interests, and this huge job of caregiving she did day after day with such joy.

Then I asked her, "Who's helping you?"

"Oh, so many people say: 'Let me know if I can help.' Or they say, 'How can I help?' But I'm doing fine, really I am."

"It's good to help the man you love. And I can see that you *are* doing a really good job, responsible for all the details of his care. Still, it may be nice to have a little help."

"My kids, the people at church, they all have their own busy lives. I don't want to bother them. They stop by after church on Sunday and visit other times and that's nice."

"And you serve them tea and cookies."

"Yes, and I enjoy it."

"Of course you do. You have a good life; I'm sure you do enjoy their visits and support and making the cookies for them. And I know you want to care for your Henry. You have to stay strong and well-rested to do that well—especially as he's getting weaker, doesn't get out of bed, and needs more from you. Likely that means you are not getting out of the house much. Full-time care of anyone can become exhausting."

"I manage."

"Absolutely, Janine, you are managing well. Still, it's important you have a break regularly so you can *keep* caring for him—and stay healthy yourself. We've found that caregivers often manage quite well for a while. Sometimes they don't want to ask for help, don't want to bother others. You've said that family, friends, neighbors, and church members often want to help—and they don't know what to do. I'd like you to think about letting others have the blessing of helping you."

"Also, it's important for your family members to take turns helping you. That's the only way they can learn what needs to be done, and realize what you do every day. When they are here and you have some time away, they can ask hospice for help and information just like you do. Show them Henry's schedule and the medications chart on the kitchen door, along with the phone number for hospice. They will feel better for having helped him and you, and they will begin to understand what you do 24/7. Your husband will benefit by having them here also."

Janine said she'd try to think of others helping as a gift they wanted to give.

"I care about you. I love your courage and the love you show. I've created a little card to help you involve your friends and church family who want to help."

Here's How You Can Help Us!

Errands and Other Help	Spend Time at Our House
(Please call first)	(Please call first)
Get groceries for us (separate sheet)	Just come by for a visit!
Walk the dog (one hour/one day/week)	Dominoes/Checkers S M T W T F S
Pharmacy run (info. on other side)	Come watch the game, date:
Mow the lawn (we have a mower)	Help me write a letter or card
Weed the flower bed	Take him/her for a drive
Bring a dessert or casserole (favorites/limitations other side)	Watch a movie together at home
Shovel the snow (we have shovels)	Read a book, newspaper, or magazine to the patient
Your idea(s):	Loan us a book or magazine
Take the kids to a movie or play date	Play cards
Patient's name:	Look at photo albums together
_____	
Home phone:	Loan a DVD
_____	
Mobile phone:	Replenish tea or coffee supply
_____	
Address:	Sit with patient so the caregiver can have time out
_____	
Directions:	Visit with a pet Your idea:
_____	_____

I gave her several copies of the cards I'd made and helped her see how to use them, explaining:

1. The card lists all kinds of things that need to be done in your home, with your husband, outside your home, or running errands for you.
2. It makes it easy for folk to choose a task, a day, and a time to help; they can do it each week or just once.
3. It shows that our hospice believes these tasks are needed regularly.
4. It lets people know really practical ways to help.
5. I've printed it on 8½" × 11" cardstock cut it in half. I'm leaving a dozen with you; let me know when you need more—or make copies.

"Taking care of your family is one of the most important things you can do. Part of my job is helping you take care of yourself. Our team wants to send a home health aide three day a week. That can give you a break too. Let me know if there are other ways we can help you stay strong physically and emotionally—and keep caring for Henry. I'll see you in a couple of weeks—and you can call hospice if you want me to come before that. Janine, you are doing such a good job!"

JACK AND CASSANDRA

Taking good care of each other.

"You'll be visiting us in our new house!" Jack said when I phoned for my first appointment with him. "Cassandra, my daughter, is taking time during her lunch hour so she can be here too."

Jack was our patient. He, his wife, daughter, son-in-law, and grandson all made huge creative adjustments in their living situations when they learned Jack was in the end stage of his lung cancer. Each family sold their home and then purchased a house together in the city, near the younger folks' work-places and school. They combined their households and settled into a large, older home ideal for this new arrangement. There were two bedrooms and a bathroom upstairs, another bedroom and bathroom downstairs back of the shared living room, dining room, kitchen, and laundry.

Jack's wife, Beth, hadn't been in on the decisions because she had advanced, but not end-stage, Alzheimer's disease. She would most likely outlive him, then the family would make new care arrangements for her after Jack died. For now, this new arrangement made their lives easier logistically and emotionally for all of them. Cassandra, her husband, and teenage son were pleased with the plan.

"Thanks for coming when we can both be here," Cassandra said when I arrived for my first visit. "Dad's so active, seems to be doing well. We sort of expect that; he's always been positive and upbeat and active," she said, hugging him. "It's hard to believe his cancer has progressed so fast. Making all these decisions about the houses, getting moved in, and now, knowing the hospice people are helping, is a wonderful solution. And it means I can concentrate on my work again," she said. "I'm nearby if they need me; my boss understands our situation and makes it as easy as possible for me."

Cassandra, Jack, and I sat at the kitchen table and had a good talk. Beth came and went, sometimes she asked a question or said something to one or all of us. Some of what she said was appropriate, some comments completely inappropriate to the situation. Once when Beth had wandered out of the kitchen, Jack said, "It's good to know the kids can help us now and figure out the best care for Beth when she needs it. For now, I'm Beth's caregiver."

I praised them for finding this wonderful solution to a difficult situation: "You've been so creative," I said. "And what a great model you are for your son and grandson."

"There were many three-generation homes in the past," Cassandra reminded us. "It's working really well. There have been lots of challenges, but we're happy."

"Jack, you've been used to being busy with a job you liked," I said. "Now you're not only retired but limited physically. Do you have hobbies? What things interest you now?"

"Well, I am doing more cooking than I did!" he said. "And I'm finding I like it! I love music, play a little ukulele and guitar, and I'm teaching my grandson to play; it's really good for both of us. Cassandra plays piano—she learned from Beth—so sometimes one or both of them join in. Beth seems to love those times. They put her in a good mood."

"Excellent! Music is such a blessing. And this is a time when you and the family can create wonderful memories. Be sure to take photos of those jam sessions and piano concerts. Make tapes, videos, or just audio recordings. Invite the neighbors! Music can be a real help to folks with Alzheimer's; sometimes it helps them to be calm and to connect with old memories. Maybe you can play songs from the eras she remembers best. Sometimes there are upsides to very difficult situations."

"I've brought you some materials that may help," I said when Beth was out of the room. "There are booklets about Alzheimer's disease and its progression, ideas for managing the changes that come to patients and to families. I really want to encourage both of you to attend one of the support groups for families of Alzheimer's patients."

Then I said, "I realize you may be dealing with personality changes in Beth—that's quite common. The frustrating thing for many spouses and children is that Alzheimer's patients can be combative, sometimes be angry, and use language they've never used before."

Jack said, "You know, we've heard about that. She is confused, she wanders, and what she says often doesn't make sense. But she doesn't get angry." They looked at each other and grinned. "It's quite a relief, actually," Cassandra said. "She's the nicest now she's been as long as I can remember!"

It was fascinating that Beth's personality shift was a positive change for her family and a reminder that each patient is unique and that the whole family is affected. There were many positives in their new complicated and difficult circumstances, and they surely were making the best of a bad situation. I believe this was the most flexible and creative family I encountered in hospice.

Chapter Four

Hospice in a Place You Call Home

Most hospice patients prefer to continue to live in their own home; when that is not possible, many creative housing and caregiving alternatives ae available:

- Living with a family member. Some hospice patients live with family members and that becomes their home. If family caregivers need to or wish to continue their employment as long as the patient is well enough, or they just want a day away from home to do errands and be with friends, community day care centers may be available.

  Some communities provide funds for a family member to be the caregiver, often requiring that they meet income, usually state Medicaid, guidelines. Homemaker or caregiver services may be available through federal, state, county, or private agencies.[1] The social worker, discharge planner, or navigator at your local hospital or the county aging and disability services office can provide information about (1) services available in your community for help at home and (2) finding a place your family member can call home.
- Community organizations in some areas provide maintenance or minor home repairs, transportation to medical appointments, and grocery services, and these communities may be the first step that can help people age fifty-five and over remain in their own home.[2]
- Co-housing communities; search the internet by state. Planning ahead is required.
- Intergenerational co-housing/on college campuses[3] and group-purchased property,[4] some including rental or leased property. Residents can have both privacy and community.
- A house purchased together where friends share the cost and space.[5]

- Retirement communities often include transition to independent and assisted living areas in the same or an adjacent building. Meals are usually included.
- Independent living facilities with assistance getting up and going to bed.
- Assisted living facilities, with personal care increased to include bathing and medications.
- Board and care homes/adult care homes with six to twelve patients. Each state has its own name and requirements for this kind of care.
- Skilled nursing facilities (SNFs). [6]

Long-term care works well in Washington state, leading all states in helping residents age in place and serving as a model for others seeking the best care available, according to a report by Larry Lipman and Dana E. Neuts in the *AARP Bulletin/Real Possibilities*, September 2017. [7]

1. Offering control over who provides personal care.
2. Answering calls for help more quickly.
3. Rebalancing Medicaid spending so more people can age at home or in the community.
4. Encouraging nursing home stays to be temporary.
5. Allowing home health aides to provide more medical care.
6. Giving family caregivers a set of instructions when patients leave the hospital.
7. Providing more housing alternatives than nursing homes.

MRS. SIMPSON

A place you call home.

The door to the ICU unit was ajar and I heard voices:

"Mom, I want to take care of you myself. I just can't."

"I know, son, I know. I've always been afraid of ending up in a nursing home. Can't we think of something?"

I knocked lightly on the unit's glass door: "Mrs. Simpson, I'm Karen, the social worker from hospice. And this is your son, Tom, right? May I talk with you both for a few minutes?"

"Yes, please come in. The hospice nurse was here earlier."

"I know you've had a lot happening recently," I began. "Your fall, your surgery, ICU. I'm so glad you've signed on to hospice. I'm here to get acquainted, answer any questions, and let you know how I can help."

"Mom's so sad," Tom said. "The doctor says he'll be releasing her soon, says she can't go back to her apartment, can't live by herself anymore. And . . ."

"The doctor says I'm not going to get better," Mrs. Simpson said quietly.

"That's hard to hear, isn't it? Is there any other family nearby who can help?"

"Tom's my only child, and I can't stay with him. My sister can't help. I guess I have to think about a nursing home. I hate that . . ."

"Can you help us with that?" Tom asked.

"Absolutely! All these changes are a lot to take in. Actually, I have some good news. I've checked with the doctor and he believes an assisted living center will be fine for you."

"I've heard about them . . ."

"You would live in your own apartment with a small kitchen; you'll likely eat one or maybe all your meals in their dining room, but you still can cook or bake if you like. The apartment is part of a larger campus, with duplexes, and a skilled nursing facility. Yep, that's a 'nursing home.' It will be there, easy to move to, if and when you need that kind of care. There are a lot of things for the active folks to do there, crafts, musical programs, and bus trips to town for shopping or movies or field trips. You'll make new friends. And medical people will help with your medications and other concerns."

"That sounds so much better than I was imagining—still, I don't think I could afford it."

"Ah, more good news," I said. "Some places charge based on your ability to pay—it's called a 'sliding scale.' And that means they would take the percentage of your income you can afford."

She already seemed calmer, less frightened. I continued: "The hospice nurses, the chaplain, and I will visit you regularly no matter where you live. Soon you'll move out of ICU to a regular hospital room, and when you're able I can take you and Tom to see some of the assisted living places nearby. How does that sound?"

They looked at each other. Mrs. Simpson said, "It sounds good. I hate not being able to go home. But I'll go see the places . . ."

"I know these are all difficult things to think about," I continued. "This kind of move is one of the hardest decisions families make, no matter how nice a place may be, no matter how safe. Thankfully, in our community, there are some really wonderful, clean, bright, and cheery places with competent and caring staff. Some of them have pets, greenhouses, craft rooms, and activity directors. There are dismal places too. The few bad ones make it hard for people to feel positive about any care facility. I'll make an appointment and we can go see a place I think you'll like when the doctor gives the okay for you to be out and about."

A few days later, Mrs. Simpson, Tom, and I visited two facilities. She made her choice. When she was discharged from the hospital, she was able to go to her apartment and oversee Tom packing up what she could take to her new apartment. If and when she moved from assisted living into a skilled nursing facility (SNF), she could choose a chair, a table and lamp, photo albums, books, a radio/CD player, TV, and plants for her room there. Some SNFs have private rooms available; some people don't want to be alone and choose to have a roommate. Sometimes there's no choice who will be room-mates. That's another huge adjustment—living with someone you don't know.

Mrs. Simpson moved to her new apartment, and eventually she did move into the SNF on the same campus. Her hospice team continued to visit her there, and she had the extra help of a hospice home health aide to supplement the SNF staff. Sometimes these facilities are better than living with family members who can't provide the care needed. They can be the safest solution for the best care.

MR. HOWARD

"I'm still here." Breathe. "Can't talk . . ." Breathe.

Mr. Howard lived in a quiet, clean, pleasant nursing home. He'd been there for many months; no family was available and he couldn't care for himself. The doctor recommended adding hospice care when his diagnosis became "end-stage emphysema." He was in a room by himself and that's what he wanted.

Each time I visited, I first checked Mr. Howard's chart and talked to the nurses to learn how he had been recently, then I walked down the hall over the squeaky-clean large black-and-white linoleum tiles to his room. Always he was sitting on the side of the bed, leaning on the bedside table, staring into the center of the room, struggling to breathe, focusing on each breath, con-nected to his lifeline, the oxygen machine, sending its regular, quiet hss-sss-ing song into the otherwise quiet room. The TV was off; I'd never seen it turned on.

"Glad to see you, Mr. Howard."

"I'm still here." *Breathe.*

He would greet me by nodding his head toward me, then purposefully taking a really deep breath. *Breathe.* Replies to my comments and queries were given in one or two words or a nod of his head. He was focused on breathing. Each breath seemed to be hard work.

"How are things today?" I asked.

"Same." *Breathe.*

"Have you thought about letting me get you a recorder and some books on tape? What kind of books do you like?"

"Thanks, honey." *Breathe.*

"I think it might help you to think about something outside this room. You might relax a bit, not be so focused on your breathing; it could even mean it would be easier to breathe."

"No, thanks." *Breathe.*

We'd "discussed" this before. Mr. Howard believed that if he concentrated on listening to a book on tape, a TV program, or the radio, he'd forget to breathe. The anatomy and physiology class I'd taken in college had convinced me that Mr. Howard's autonomic nervous system's reaction to his not taking a breath would remember for him. It's actually hard to *not* breathe. And if or when he did stop breathing, the oxygen machine alarm would let the nurses at the station know there was a problem and come to help. His anxiety likely even made his breathing harder. I tried to explain that to him, but he didn't believe me—or want to hear it again.

He told me he feared that, when he went to sleep and wasn't focusing on the breathing, he would stop breathing and not wake up. He was ill enough that it was possible he would die in the night, so I didn't try to convince him otherwise. I just wanted him to be less fearful. What he wanted was to focus on his breathing, believing that his job was to concentrate on breathing. He wanted no distractions.

It was truly amazing to me how he could adapt to that limited life. When I suggested things to enrich his life, he said breathing was enough "quality of life" for him at this point. Our team had shared ideas on how to help and decided we would honor his choices. Still, I kept trying to find ways to help. I couldn't help it; it's where my mind goes when I see a problem: "fix it."

"I'd love to hear about the work you did before you retired, Mr. Howard."

"Can't . . ." *Breathe.*

"I wish we could do a mind-meld and I could learn it from you—even in that way."

He grinned; that seemed like a new thought to him. "That's nice, thanks." *Breathe.*

"You must have seen and experienced so many interesting things in your long life."

"Yep. And some . . ." *Breathe.* ". . . not so nice."

"May I read to you? What did you use to read—novels, Westerns, romance?"

That got a wider grin, and then he said, "Chaplain reads." *Breathe.* "That's enough." "Anything you'd like me to do here before I leave—or something I can do for you out there in the outside world," I asked, smiling and raising my eyebrows as if I really expected to hear something I could do to help him. He and I knew he wouldn't have any requests, but I think he enjoyed my trying.

"Nope." *Breathe.*

"Okay. Be sure to have the nurses call me if you think of something or just want to talk—anytime."

I winked at him after that last statement. He grinned and took another breath. He may have wanted to talk, or maybe he never was a talker. Every waking moment he focused on his breathing, on every breath. It was exhausting to watch. As I stood to leave, Mr. Howard looked up, focused on my eyes, and held me there for a moment with these words:

"I know . . ." *Breathe.* ". . . you want to help me." *Breathe.* "Thanks."

Then he turned his eyes down at the bedside table and dismissed me gently with the statement: "Tired." *Breathe.*

He'd had enough company and talking and listening for today; he wanted me to leave. I put my hand gently on his shoulder—I'd already learned he didn't want a hug—and I left. I walked over those big black-and-white linoleum tiles back to the nurses' station, wrote my sad notes on his chart, went out the door to my car, and got in. I just sat for a while, sad for him, wishing I knew better how to help. Perhaps just being there for him regularly, the gentle jokes, the wanting to help was enough. Then I drove away. He was okay being sort of alone—in his own room—with nurses and meds nearby, and his visits from hospice caregivers.

SUSAN JOHNSON

Multiple diagnoses, needing an advocate.

One of the most delicate parts of my job was advocating for patients in skilled nursing homes (SNFs). We wanted a good partnership with the administration and staff, and we needed to be sensitive to patients' unmet needs and report them. Our hospice nurses saw our SNF patients at least twice a week, working with the SNF nursing staff and managing decisions about their meds relating to their terminal diagnosis and extra equipment needed; our aides helped patients three to five days a week as extra hands and extra care, in addition to the busy SNF staff. I visited every week or two, and the hospice nurse and I met in a staff meeting with the SNF nurses about once a month.

Susan Johnson was a nursing home resident when she came onto our hospice program. Her cancer had progressed, and no further treatment for a cure was advisable. In addition, she had advanced rheumatoid arthritis and, one more thing, advanced Parkinson's disease. Her joints ached and were stiff; she had tremors in her hands and very limited speech. She could do almost nothing for herself.

"Hi, Mrs. Johnson, I'm Karen. I'm part of your hospice team, the social worker," I introduced myself on my first visit. "May I come in?" She nodded affirmatively. She was lovely, with snow white hair and a warm smile in her eyes.

"I'm happy to meet you. I'm sorry you're having so many difficulties—cancer, rheumatoid arthritis and some pain, Parkinson's." *More nodding and smiling. No words.* I continued: "It's my understanding that when people have Parkinson's disease they usually understand very well what's said to them." *Nodding.* "Also, I'm told that sometimes it's very difficult to get out just the right words—so you may not talk very much." *Vigorous nodding!*

I stood near the bed and put my hand on her arm. Her smile brightened and there were tears in the corners of her bright blue eyes seeming to signal a kind of relief. She believed somebody understood why she didn't talk much. I asked questions she could answer with simple gestures or nods. Her knuckles were enlarged, her fingers bent down, contracted. I thought about how difficult it would be to push a button to get attention from the staff. *How does she ask for medication or a drink or to have the TV turned down or off?*

She seemed to enjoy my visit. The TV was on and I asked her if that was okay with her. She nodded—and I know open-ended questions are the best, but in this situation, I tried to anticipate what would be helpful and important to her. "Would you like the TV turned off?" She indicated a "No . . ." by closing her eyes and turning her head from side to side. I said, "Ah, maybe it's company?" She nodded her head in the affirmative. "Can you hear it alright . . . ?" and my Q and A and her physical reactions continued.

Her roommate was silent because she was semi-comatose. Often nursing home administrators arrange for an alert patient to have a roommate who is silent—almost like having a private room! "It must be a lonely life—difficult to talk, your roommate doesn't talk at all. I'll bet some of the nurse aides are friendly and try to communicate." She gave me a small sweet and expressive smile. The SNF aides do most of the personal care and they are very busy. "I'm glad our hospice nurse and nurse aide are also helping," I said. "She nodded agreement."

On my next visit, Mrs. Johnson seemed to be in pain. I went back to the nurses' station and asked if she could have some pain meds. They checked the chart and took her meds to her. I usually visited her once a week to "talk." Each time I'd read the nurses notes, visit her, find she needed pain meds, and go back to the nurses' station, ask for meds, and we'd wait for the decision whether it was "time yet" for her meds.

I noted that in the list of diagnoses on her chart, number one (the primary diagnosis) was "drug-seeking behavior" and vowed to talk to our team about it. We would discuss it and make necessary recommendations that the more serious diagnoses were listed first when we had our regular meeting with the nursing home staff.

During one visit I remember asking if she could have the pain medication already ordered, the nurse told me, "Well, she hasn't asked for any."

My response: "She's indicated to me that she's in pain. Rheumatoid ar-thritis makes it impossible for her to move her thumb to push her call bell. Unless someone is in the room and asks her, or if she is sometimes able to ask, how do you know what she wants? Please check . . ."

"I'll see . . ." she said, and I tried to accept that nurses are only there one shift at a time; they have many patients and cannot always remember the special needs of each patient. Communication between the aides and nurses is vital, especially with patients with very limited communication skills. I tried to be patient and think how to keep this from happening again.

Back in Mrs. Johnson's room, we visited and waited. While I was decid-ing what to do next to get her the meds now, Jan, our hospice nurse, arrived. I told her what was happening and she did a thorough exam. One of Susan's toes was swollen, purple, and the nail was barely attached.

I asked Susan what happened and she quietly said, ". . . the aide. . . ."

Our hospice nurse and I looked at each other, and Jan went into action, walking to the station to report the incident to the nurses and asking for her pain meds. They agreed that this would be discussed at the next nursing home/hospice team meeting. Jan came back to the room, gently repaired the nail, and bandaged it. Sometimes a patient may not complain about the person (the aide) who causes something like a damaged toe—the patient still has to rely on that aide for most of the care she receives. The SNF adminis-tration was responsive and disciplined the aide.

Another day I stopped in Susan's doorway holding, on the upturned flat of my hand like a waiter, a pot of red geraniums. "Now, why would I bring you flowers today?" I asked, sort of to the room in general. Usually, her only response was a smile. Today she said, clearly, "Because it's the birthday of a very important person."[8]

"Fabulous! You said a whole sentence. Good for you!" She beamed.

What joy for both of us! I put the flower on the windowsill near her bed. Haltingly, she had told me that she loved to look out her window, remember-ing her own backyard in her own home, talking about her flowers and the birds she'd seen at her feeders.

It was fortunate that I visited her on another day when Medicare review-ers were in the nursing home. I went to the room where they were working on a stack of charts and asked if I could have Susan Johnson's chart to read the notes and enter my own.

"She may not be able to stay on hospice, not if Diagnosis No. 1 is 'drug-seeking behavior,'" the reviewer said. That would mean she still would be in the nursing facility but without the oversight of our nurse, the extra care from our home health aide, and visits from the rest of the team.

I explained that our hospice team and the nursing home staff had agreed that the order would be changed to reflect reality as hospice saw it: No. 1. Cancer, end stage; No. 2. Parkinson's disease, end stage; No. 3. Rheumatoid arthritis, advanced. The nursing home staff could add "drug-seeking behavior" as diagnosis 4 if they wished.

Our team helped her through the last few months of her life, working with the SNF team to provide the best care. Anyone can report concerns about patient care to the advocates or ombudsmen available through the regulatory offices in each state.

JANET

Alone and okay with that!

Janet wanted a roommate with her in the nursing home. She didn't talk to her roommate very much, or to anyone else, but she wanted someone there. Janet had a spinal deformity, could not walk, and could not get in and out of bed by herself. She could move herself about a bit once she was helped into her wheelchair. She also had chronic lung disease and had been limited physically as long as she could remember. Her mental ability was also limited; in addition, she'd gone to school only through the fifth grade. She had lived with her mother until a few years earlier; then her mother died and there were no siblings to help. No one even came to visit her. Still, she seemed quite contented with her limited activities, her life, and her care. Her interests were as limited as her abilities—she watched TV and looked at magazines. Many times when I visited her, our conversation began the same way:

"Ready for a drive, Janet?" I'd ask.

"Oh, yes. Can we go to Whataburger?"

"That's what I was thinking," I'd say.

"I'd like a Whataburger, Jr. They're small, like me, just my size."

I visited her regularly. The visits weren't long because there wasn't much she wanted to talk about or learn. Sometimes we drove to Whataburger; sometimes I just purchased the burgers for us both and we ate them in her room. I brought her magazines, offered books from the library, and offered to arrange for books on tape. She was not interested. She said she was satisfied with her life. She was safe, she had caring people around her, and she was content.

Her lung problems worsened; the nursing home decided to admit her to the hospital. Even through that decision and the move, there was no drama. There seemed to be no regrets. I went with her, and we talked a bit there. I stayed with her in the hospital on her last afternoon and into the evening; part of the time she let me hold her hand. I told her it had been good to be her friend. She didn't want to talk, didn't want me to say much. She did want me to stay, and, just before morning, still holding my hand, she died as peacefully as she had lived.

It's important to be able to offer help and then accept people and their lives just as they wish them to be. We don't have to understand; sometimes we just need to be there.

MS. CYNTHIA

The Classy Hat Lady.

I always looked forward to my visits with Ms. Cynthia. The place she now called home was a lovely skilled nursing facility in a small town. We had many good talks about her life, her family, her work, her joys, and the concerns she had now. She made friends in the facility, and her son visited her frequently. Physically, she was declining, but said she was comfortable, secure with the extra help from our nurses; emotionally, she was joyful even though there was a sure decline in her health. It was a delight to spend time with her. She knew she wouldn't survive her congestive heart failure much longer. We had good talks about her travel-filled life.

Her private room was decorated with her own stylish, beautiful lamps, an antique rocker, curved-leg side table, and lovely antique dresser topped with elegant bottles of perfume. There were many meaningful things in her room that she treasured from her past. She was classy and fabulous as Coco Chanel is reported to have said a woman should be.

There was a hat rack filled with beautiful and fun hats that she wore now and then. I love hats and she urged me to try on some of hers. There was one I especially loved, a finely woven black straw beauty with a brim you could turn up, down, or at a jaunty angle.

Ms. Cynthia learned I would be attending meetings in Chicago. She talked about the times she'd been in Chicago, the things she had seen and done there, the shops, the restaurants, and the Art Institute. We both loved that town. She said she'd almost feel like she was getting one more trip if I'd wear her lovely black straw hat to Chicago. And she said if I did that, she'd want me to have the hat as a keepsake. What a classy woman, intelligent, still curious about life and what was going on in the world. She was full of mental energy and gentle kindness.

She asked me to promise I'd wear the hat on the trip and I did: I wore it on the plane going to Chicago and in the lovely restaurant in Printer's Row, but not to my meetings. My trip was more fun because of her; I sort of felt her beside me.

A few weeks later, her hospice nurse and I arrived at the convalescent center in time to be with Ms. Cynthia and her son for a few hours during her passing. We spent time with him after she'd peacefully closed her eyes for the last time, and he shared wonderful family memories. That was a really excellent nursing home, providing good care, encouraging each resident or his or her family to fill the room with as much personality as possible. They allowed privacy and also had many ways for the residents to be active together when they wanted that. They helped make the end of life the best it could be.

Ms. Cynthia's positive attitude about life and her realistic look at her coming death remind me of Norman Lear's attitude. He was part of a B-27 bomber crew in World War II, a novice press agent and sketch writer for Jerry Lewis and Danny Thomas, and then an extremely successful writer and producer. Some of his life had been hard, and he did not want to die, but he titled his memoir: *Even This I Get to Experience.*[9]

Many choices other than the patient's own home:
Adult day care including noon meal. Pay by the hour, day or week.
Meals on Wheels & Emergency Alert System when patient is alone.
Apartment or room in the home of a family member.
Respite care by the day or week while family is on vacation.
Retirement community which may include the following choices:
Apartment with assisted living benefits (e.g., help with meditation, some or all meals)
Duplex or condominium with assisted living benefits in adjacent center.
Convalescent center or nursing home; often with specialized memory care units.
Group home (usually four to eight residents)
Hospice facility

****

All the above may be available using private pay or on a sliding scale, VA or Medicaid benefits.

Hospice and facility social workers and administrators will assist with financial arrangements.

Check it out:
Call for a personal tour and/or view video online.
Stop in unannounced for a visit; talk to other residents.
Licensed health advocates may be available in your community.
Advocates or ombudsmen are available in each state.
www.SeniorGuidebook.com; local experts covering senior issues.
www.PatientPower.info; audio and video medical info programming.

Chapter Five

Finding Meaning

Ideally, people find meaning and joy in their relationships with friends and family, their education, work, travel, belief systems, and service. Memories of those things bring special satisfaction. It was fascinating to me and helpful to patients to find ways to bring to mind and talk about special memories, things that gave their lives meaning and purpose. Some were private, shared just between us, and many they shared with their caregivers and other family members, including small children. Some of them I can share here.

Many of my patients had "visited" the Philippines when they were in the service in World War II. My family and I lived there for three years under martial law during the Marcos regime, so that connection helped as I talked with some of my patients about their military experience. I learned that some of them had never told their families anything about that time. All military experience changes a person; sometimes they want to talk about it, sometimes they don't.

Viktor Frankl, the neurologist and psychiatrist, was twenty-eight years old when he was taken prisoner by the Germans in 1942. He survived physically and emotionally. His book *Man's Search for Meaning*[1] offers a very positive, encouraging exploration about how focusing on the things that give their lives meaning continues to gives people strength and courage.

Caregivers and health care professionals find meaning in helping to make the lives of their patients less stressful and more comfortable. Public health researcher, Robert Buckingham, PhD, one of the founding fathers of the hospice movement, reports that hospice patients have less anxiety, better social adjustment, and pain control than non-hospice patients.[2]

When the here and now is difficult, finding meaning in good memories, past stories, and meaningful accomplishments helps the patient and the family become closer and focus on the value of being together in the present.

LIFE REVIEW IDEAS

There are many ways to encourage helpful remembering: photo albums, family videos, and songs can all trigger memories. Ask questions and enjoy the memories together. You can even make a video of the memory time, and photos from albums and music can be incorporated into the video—or just keep it in your heart forever. Here are some open-ended questions that can help get the conversations started:

> Tell me a favorite childhood memory. What was your favorite game or song?
>
> Tell me about your parents. Where did they come from? What kind of work did they do?
>
> Tell me about your favorite teacher. What were your favorite subjects?
>
> What did you do for Christmas, Thanksgiving, and your birthday when you were a child?
>
> Who are some of the important people from your childhood, your school days?
>
> How did you meet mom (or dad)?
>
> What sports did you like to play?
>
> Tell me what you've heard about your family before they came to America.
>
> What cities and states have you visited?
>
> What was your most enjoyable job? What would you like to create?
>
> Tell me about your favorite vacation. What's on your Bucket List?
>
> Tell me about the countries you have visited and about where you've been in America.
>
> What do you think God/Allah/Jehovah/The Great Spirit is like?
>
> Did you ever want to be a priest/preacher/imam/rabbi?
>
> What do you want me to tell my kids about you?
>
> What's the most important thing you ever learned?
>
> What things mean the most to you?

See "A Guide for Recalling and Telling Your Life Story" for more help.[3]

MR. ROBERTS, MR. SAUNDERS, AND MARTIN

"I was there . . . I served my country."

Mr. Roberts stretched his arms out in front of him across the kitchen table, his elbows touching the Formica top, his hands floating just a few inches above it, reaching toward me. Forcefully he slapped his hands together—over and over: *Crack! Crack! Crack! Crack!*

Startled, his daughter and I jumped—surprised, wondering. Then *Crack! Crack! Crack!* he did it again. It was a jarring sound, obviously very meaningful to him.

"That's the sound of bullets hitting canteens, guns," he said. "When they hit the men, there was often a soft *thud* sound."

He closed his eyes, tilted his chin up like he was listening, and said, "I can imagine it right now, feel the sand under me like I was with my buddies on that Normandy beach during the landing. When the bullets hit the sand, they made a strange *swishing* sound and stayed there to remind us of what was happening and that one could have struck us."

He was quiet for a few seconds, then: "Tuesday, the 6th of June, 1944, D-Day. Thousands of us . . . all petrified."

Reports give the number of Allied soldiers who landed on the beaches that day as 160,000. The sounds stayed with him; the *Crack!* of the guns, the cries of soldiers, the metal grinding on sand as the landing craft came close to shore to unload the men. The sounds and the sight of dead soldiers haunted him. He told us, "They say somewhere between 4,000 and 6,000[4] of them died that day."

Mr. Roberts continued talking about the smells of sulfur and blood, more sounds of grenades and screams; some sights he didn't want to describe to us. But he *did* want to tell us about that amazing and frightening experience. He told us that for years there were times he recalled the sounds, sights, and odors in his dreams—and there were times when he was awake that his mind would become crowded with the memories.

Of course, he had good memories too, of the friends he'd made, the interesting places he'd traveled to, and of serving his country. His travels were still vivid to him.

"Before the war, I'd never been outta Texas."

Veterans have so much to share; it's fascinating to listen to their memories of traveling to far-off places. My family and I lived in the Philippines from 1978 to 1981 while my husband was there to teach; now many of my patients were veterans who told me they had "visited" there too. That was a helpful point of contact between myself and them; a place to start talking about meaningful things in their lives. Some men had brought objects back from their travels that they wanted to show me; many wanted to describe what they'd experienced. Those things said forcefully, "I was there. I endured that. I served my country. I survived."

Memories of the most meaningful events in a life, especially those we are most proud of, can bring real fulfillment and peace. Some veterans just wanted to say they had served; many did not want to say more. The experience of being in a war changes a person dramatically inside, beginning with the training that really resocializes them, normalizing things they never thought they would have to learn about or do. Some had not wanted to go; some had been eager to be in the military, to serve. All told me they were proud to have served, even when there were regrets for specific actions. They did what they had to do. Arriving in a country new to them was a profound culture shock. Coming home was a "reverse culture shock"; many did not want to talk of any of it again, and some talked about it lot.

I remember the looks on the faces of some spouses or children, silently begging me to please not let their father or grandfather get started on "that war stuff." They acted as if they had heard it too often. When that happened, I talked to the veteran when the family wasn't around. Other times, adults and children were transfixed listening to their granddad's or dad's stories. Some of them, Mr. Roberts's daughter included, had never heard the stories before I was there and asked them about their military experience.

Another veteran I remember fondly was Mr. Saunders, a widower living with his son, daughter-in-law, and grandchildren in their quiet, pleasant home in the country. The family greeted me warmly; we chatted a bit altogether, then the family said they'd like Mr. Saunders to have time to talk privately with me. They left us alone in a sort of family room/sickroom where they made him the center of attention and care. He was very ill. He lay quietly in his hospital bed, his small hands holding the covers pulled up to his chin, speaking softly and slowly. We were comfortably talking about his life in general, and then he said he wanted to tell me about his military experience. He seemed to *need* to talk about it.

Mr. Saunders was a gentle man who had done things he didn't like to remember but needed to talk about. He said he was proud of his service but so disgusted by much of what he had seen, and he told me about some of it. I wish I'd gotten permission to record our conversation so I could have shared it with his son. Mr. Saunders died the very next day.

When I talked with his family later, sharing some of the things about his war experience that he'd given me permission to tell them, they told me he'd never told them any of it. They were happy to know how his own personal military experience had been such a meaningful part of his life and that he'd been able to tell someone.

My father-in-law, Martin, was proud of his service in the Civilian Conservation Corps (CCC)[5] in the 1930s. We'd heard many of his stories, learning about their work to create public parks and monuments. In the last few months of his life, he responded to our usual questions and comments, but he was not beginning many conversations. However, when I began this sentence, "Dad, it was really wonderful, wasn't it, to be part of the CCC . . ." he was always eager to tell us the CCC stories and share the memories, often with a breaking voice and tears in his eyes.

Those activities had allowed him to work in the woods of Michigan, which he loved. The country was improved through the efforts of the CCC and similar U.S. programs, and the workers had meaningful work during the years after the Great Depression. It was an important involvement for citizens and he was so proud to have been part of that. It mattered a great deal to him. He loved those memories and his chance to be of service to America. He wanted us to know and he loved remembering and telling us. It was one of the things that added meaning to his life.

EMILY AND CHARLES

"Tell me your story."

Meaning in Stories

Emily and Charles raised a family together; he'd had a successful business career, she had focused on their home and children. Her joy was homemaking cooking, baking, childcare, decoration—she said she even enjoyed the cleaning required to make it all beautiful. He retired and they fished together, worked in the yard, and watched old movies; they were thoroughly enjoying their years of retirement. Then Charles became gravely ill, and when he came onto our hospice program, he was already bedfast and comatose.

Emily insisted that his hospital bed be in the living room, asking folks who visited to talk to him a bit. He didn't answer. He hardly moved at all. Emily loved to tell us the stories of their life together. She wanted to tell those stories in the living room, just in case he could hear and enjoy her reminiscences. Daily she rubbed his immobile limbs with cocoa cream, gave him his meds, and reminded him of the stories of their life together. We expected and she *knew* he was content with the care. They were still "being there" for each other.

Meaning in Things

Near the end of my mom's life, she spent a lot of time resting on the living room sofa. One afternoon I asked if there was some project I could do for her, and she said: "You know, I've been meaning to clean out that blue cabinet."

I happily sat on the floor in front of that cabinet of treasures, a buffet my dad had antiqued; I opened the doors to the lower two shelves, taking out the lovely dishes one at a time. That day we both enjoyed looking at her antique china and other treasures.

"I love looking at these beautiful things," I said to her. "Tell me about them. . . . Where did you get this one?" And for a couple of hours, we talked about the stories connected with some of our shared histories and I tidied up the collection.

Occasionally she said, "You love that bowl, please take it. I don't use it anymore. I want you to have it." Ah, I'd known this was coming, we both knew it was a part of saying goodbye, and she made it easy. That afternoon we didn't talk about her illness, we talked about our memories, and she loved giving me things precious to us both. Now, I have the blue cabinet and I often think about that lovely afternoon and the precious time with my mom.

When visiting my patients, I often asked about interesting objects in their home—artifacts, collections, china, curiosities. I was truly interested in those things; I'd considered being an anthropologist because of my interest in cultures and artifacts. I learned a lot from listening to the stories that followed my asking about the things—and those things took patients back in thought to times and places meaningful to them.

Often things are connected to meaningful and important events in the lives of their owners, and sometimes they involved their travels. When I complimented one of our patients on her cabinet full of lovely "Thousand Flowers" china, she shared her memories of her travel to Japan and her love of anything Japanese. I told her I understood and I had a small tea set of that same design that I treasured from my visit to Japan.

By my front door is a ceramic umbrella stand with an Asian design. In it are umbrellas and canes. When visitors ask about the canes, I have stories to share—one cloisonné cane belonged to my mother-in-law, one black gnarled walking stick is from my husband's grandfather, and there are walking sticks made by my husband for our grandchildren. There's a heavy wooden cane from a hospice patient who hand-carved canes for himself, his family, and friends, and he gave me one. Each of those things has special meaning for me; I treasure them and the part they played in my life. One day I'll tell my daughter, son, or grandchildren the stories of each one. One day they will own them.

Meaning in Spiritual Belief

"My son was baptized in a river in the Philippines," a gentleman told me when he learned that we had also lived there for several years. We were looking through his photo album and he described the scene—tropical greenery, a river, people in the river in robes.

"Fascinating, tell me more . . ." The retired missionary shared many things about living and working in another culture. That was a huge and important period in his life. It seemed to really help him to talk about it. It was a way to remember some things that still gave meaning to his life. I loved sharing the story of our son's baptism in a river in the Philippines, and we marveled at the connections in our lives.

Spiritual belief and religion play a major role in the lives of the majority of human beings. Each hospice has social workers, chaplains, sometimes called spiritual guides, available to talk about the beliefs and spiritual things that provide meaning to their clients. In addition, it's vital that all the hospice personnel be open, listen to, and support what a person believes about ultimate things. The end of life is a time for reaffirming belief, not a time for proselytizing.

"People live and die by drawing on the spiritual resources that have been passed down to them from mentors in life and faith," writes John Fanestil. In *Mrs. Hunter's Happy Death* he describes the concept, popular in the mid-1800s, of anticipating a "happy death" made possible by focusing on spiritual peace. [6]

Our Stories of Meaning Say: "I Was Here, and It Matters"

For each person, what matters, what "means" to us, involves thinking of what we have accomplished, the impact that things and people have had on our lives: parents, partners, children, friends, education, work, religion, music, art, travel. It's helpful to review meaningful events and memories, reminding us that "I was here, and it matters." Thinking about those meaningful things between diagnosis and death can actually lead to spiritual growth.

One special blessing of hospice is being part of helping the patient and their partners, family members, and friends take the time to remember and talk about the meaningful people and events in their lives. See the ideas at the beginning of this chapter for ways to help folks tell their stories and remember the meaningful events in their lives.

After a death occurs, stories continue to help family members talk about meaningful memories. Many hospices offer annual services to families to remember the folk who have passed. The Providence Hospice of Seattle calls their annual memorial service "Stories of the Heart." Our hospice also had an annual event to honor our patients and their families, and that was very meaningful to us; community members were invited also.

JERRY

Memories . . . a winding road, a river, and a song.

When I think of Jerry, three things come to mind: a long winding road, an unusual river, and a song. The drive from our hospice office to Jerry's place took me about forty-five minutes, but the road I particularly remember was the one from the highway to his home. It was long, winding, and beautiful, including a lovely wooded area, mostly oaks, before reaching his yard where there were several colorful lawn chairs, a fire pit, and quiet surroundings. It seemed a peaceful place. The river is a bit harder to describe.

First, it's important to know about Jan, Jerry's wife. She had died within a few days of being admitted to our hospice program and I had never met her. We were always sad when our patients had "a short stay," wishing we could have offered them care and attention for a longer period of time, ideally the full six months hospice offers. Soon after she passed, we learned in our team meeting that, when he drove his wife to the hospital that last time, Jerry already knew that *he* had a tumor on his neck. After Jan had her surgery, he took her home from the hospital and they had a few precious days together before she died in their bed. A few days after her funeral, Jerry had surgery to remove *his* tumor; soon after he was told it was malignant and very advanced. Now *he* was our patient.

How can one man manage so much in such a short time? Often, when I've felt things were piling up in my life with too many difficult things too close together, I would think: *This is too hard; it's not fair.* My son tells me: "Fair is that thing that happens once a year south of Dallas with Big Tex greeting you by the front gate." He was referring to the State Fair of Texas. When things become difficult in my life, sometimes I think of Jerry.

"You better prepare yourself," Jerry's hospice nurse had warned me, and she'd explained: "Because of where the tumor was, and how large it was, the surgery was dramatic and extensive. Now the wound looks sort of like a 'river' running along the side of his neck. The wound is draining and we have to keep it open. You can't see it that much looking at him from the front. You'll be alright. I just wanted you to know before you met him."

My mind was on "the river" and my heart was already full when Jerry opened the door that first time I met him. He was a big guy with a gentle demeanor; one of the calmest and most pleasant people I've ever known. After the initial greetings, we sat down at his lovely round, oak kitchen table. He offered me sweet tea, and he seemed quite matter of fact about his life. We had a good talk. It was very pleasant there with the door open and birds singing outside. With most of my attention focused on Jerry's face, I still saw a bit of that "river" and I said, "I'm so sorry you're having to deal with so many difficult things. First, how is the wound?"

"You know, it's really not much of a bother. The nurse is great, keeps it clean and tells me how to manage. And it doesn't hurt."

"I understand that the nurses have things under control; what a blessing. Now tell me what you'd like to share about your wife—I'm so sorry about her death."

He described their marriage as a real joy, especially because they felt it was so delightful to have found each other after each had experienced previous bad relationships. The only thing that seemed really difficult for Jerry to talk about was "the song," but he wanted to share that part of their story too. He and his wife loved listening to Barbra Streisand, one song in particular.

Jerry said, "The song 'Places that Belong to You' was our favorite. It reminded us, reminds me, of our lives. May I play it for you now? We can talk about it and more about her later, but right now we just need to listen . . ."

We sat quietly and listened to the words and music, tears in our eyes. Each of us thinking about the meaning of the words for ourselves—and I imagined what they must mean to Jerry.

The words seemed perfect for his story.

"That was our song," he said. "It was playing on the radio when I drove her to the hospital the last time."

So there was the "long winding road" and that "unusual river" and "the song."

During our second talk we sat in Jerry's peaceful yard under the trees and Jerry talked about his childhood home, his family, his career, his first marriage, the joy of his life with Jan—and his feelings about having no children. He said he was at peace because he believes he and Jan will be together again. Then he asked me something that touched me so deeply that it stays with me during my difficult times.

He asked, "How are *you*? Who sings for the songbird?"

Here was another allusion to Streisand's magic with words and music. Tears came to my eyes. What I did was often difficult, being present, listening, empathizing, helping when I could, and not letting their stories take over my life. Still, things did pile up and I thanked Jerry for looking into my heart and mind, for being concerned about me. How kind.

I don't even know how many funerals I attended in my time with hospice. I went to the services whenever I could, to honor my patients and their families, wanting to help others process life and death. Because of Jerry's life, his kindness, and his sensitivity, I came undone at Jerry's funeral; Marty, our chaplain, noticed and came to stand with me, his hand on my shoulder. Then I remembered Jerry's calmness about his dying, his surety, not understanding how, but believing he'd be with his wife soon. I gained control of my emotions, wiped the tears away, and was calmed by my memories of him. He believed the story and the song would continue. Still, tears come to my eyes again each time I think of Jerry's story and his kindness to me.

Chapter Six

Dramatic Challenges

Hospice patients and caregivers experience many negative feelings—sadness, anger, anxiety, and fear—due to the patient's diagnosis, physical and emotional changes, or limitations. Their emotional pathway may move from disappointment to discouragement, sometimes to despair and depression. They may fear they'll not be able to manage. Usually, when hospice personnel become involved, physical and emotional stresses become more manageable. Support from people trained to help relieves some of the challenges of facing a life-limiting illness.

For some, there are serious challenges. They may feel desperate or threaten harm to themselves or others. It is vital that each hospice team member have training in recognizing the signs of desperation, complicated grief, and/or depression, develop skills so they can communicate with persons who are severely troubled, and report these concerns to the team. A clear understanding of when and how to notify authorities when a person is a danger to themselves or others is vital. There also needs to be a well-thought-out weapons policy, clearly understood by the team, the patient, the caregiver, and other family members.

Our hospice experienced one suicide while I was on the team. A gun was the implement and the death occurred within the first few days after the patient and his wife signed onto hospice care. The nurse and I arrived on the scene within an hour of the event. We spent time with his wife and waited for other family members to arrive. Each of us spent time with her at the funeral and in the days following. She was fortunate to have a supportive family nearby, neighbors who assisted her, and a pastor who assured her. He told her not to assume that the patient could not go to heaven. She needed to hear that; his explanation was that God understands that there are life events that a person cannot handle. That conversation with her pastor gave her great comfort.

Suicidal thoughts are said to be "common among hospice patients"; however, reports are uncommon in the literature [1] and in the media. I believe there are several reasons:

1. The initial assessments and ongoing evaluations by the hospice team often identify when a crisis is building and address it.
2. Patients receive immediate attention to symptom control and are more comfortable physically, which makes emotional comfort more likely.
3. In states where "death with dignity/patient-assisted suicide" is legal, patients who make that choice may also request hospice care. Hospice personnel offer nonjudgmental support; patients need to talk with hospice representatives and verify their guidelines about "death with dignity/patient-assisted suicide."
4. In newspapers and other media, reporting of suicide and/or details may be suppressed. The only suicide I was able to identify in newspapers online was a murder/suicide in which a spouse killed the patient and then himself. Guidelines for the media [2] advise caution in reporting, not sensationalizing the story, and providing information about phone numbers and websites about suicide prevention is always a part of the reporting.

MINNIE AND JACK

"I want just the two of us to talk."

Minnie was busy preparing our coffee when I arrived for a visit. The sugar bowl and creamer were already on the table, and our cups and saucers were waiting there for us too. As usual, she was talking nonstop, sharing neighborhood gossip. Minnie and Jack knew almost everyone in the mobile home park where they lived and kept track of them all. Gregarious Jack knew most everybody there and lots of folks in town too.

When there was a bit of a hiatus in her delightful descriptions of people and events, I said, "Minnie, what a fun dish," indicating an eight-inch light green ceramic bowl sitting on the top of her refrigerator. It was shaped like a cabbage. "Where did you get that?"

"That old thing? I don't even remember. Do you like it? Take it."

"Oh, my, I didn't mean I want it," I said, frustrated with myself for not remembering how to admire something in another person's home. You'd think I'd learned that well enough in the three years we'd lived in the Far East; there, if you indicate that you admire something, the owner is obliged to give it to you. I had learned to say something like "What a beautiful vase—it looks so pretty there where you have it with that flower in it." Then the owner could keep it because it was perfect where it was. I do own a few special possessions that show I didn't always remember how to properly give a compliment there either.

"But you like it," Minnie said. "Can't remember where I got it, don't even use it—doesn't mean a thing to me. Take it." And I now own a beautiful old light green eight-inch cabbage-shaped ceramic bowl. My employer allowed me to receive and keep gifts if the value was under $25. I always think of Minnie when I see it or use it. It's a delightful, meaningful memory of our friendship and this family's complicated story.

Minnie was a tiny woman with an "in-your-face" directness. Attempting to be as culturally correct as possible, I asked her if I should call her a Native American, American Native, or First Nations woman. "I'm Injun," she'd said, very proud of her heritage.

She had lived in Seattle with her first husband. Most of her Washington family worked in the fish canneries. She enjoyed sharing those memories, and the stories were fascinating to me because I too had lived and raised a family in Washington state. We talked about her marriage, her children, her son who was in prison, and Justin, her grandson, now living with them. Then she talked about meeting Jack.

Minnie had end-stage lung cancer, and soon after we began caring for her she became quite fragile and grudgingly agreed to spend most of her time in the hospital bed we provided. We set it up in the small, narrow living room in their mobile home, and that became the center of her world. When she got up to go to the back of the trailer to the bathroom, she almost never took her medical alert device with her. "I'm just goin' back to the bathroom," she'd say.

"Minnie, this little button is for you to call for help if you fall—*on your way* to the bathroom! This cord is so you'll wear it around your neck *all the time*, to be safer."

"I'm not gonna fall; I have those walls to hang on to." *You can lead a horse to water, but* . . . I thought each time I visited and told her the same thing.

Jack was big, boisterous, and loud, often teasing and making jokes. "So why do you spend all this time with Minnie?" he asked me one day. "I never get to talk to you by myself."

"Ah, Jack, you walked right into that one," I shot back. "Next time I come, I'll meet you for breakfast in town. I want just the two of us to talk—in public, of course."

"Oh, you got me. I don't have much to talk about 'cause I know what *you* want to talk about. But I'd love to be seen in public with you," Jack flirted. Minnie groaned. I smiled.

One morning I met Jack at his favorite breakfast place in town; he was his boisterous, loud, and charming self. He knew 'most everybody there, and whenever someone entered the restaurant, he called out to them:

"This is Karen, she's my social worker from hospice. She's psychologizin' me."

Of course, it wasn't easy to talk about anything of substance in the middle of that very public restaurant—but we had a pleasant time together, and Jack began to feel more at ease with me. After that, it was easier for us to find a few minutes to talk about things of substance when I was at their home. And sometimes just a sentence could help him share his feelings.

One day I said, "Some people believe there are four basic feelings: being sad or mad or glad or scared.[3] You know like 'glad it's sunny today instead of raining' or 'mad the dog's feet dirtied your carpet.'"

Jack said, "I'm mad she's so sick. And I'm scared . . ." Then we could talk about what scared him.

Minnie was very open about everything in her life. Sometimes she would talk about being mad that she couldn't "do for folks" anymore. And she was mad and sad about her son Clay who was in prison. "Nothin' scares me anymore; hell, I've been through so much. And I'm tired—just maybe scared what will happen to Justin."

Justin was sixteen, attending high school, being a normal teenager. They felt very protective of him. He had many conflicting emotions because he cared about each person in that complicated family drama. Minnie and Jack wanted what was best for him, but really didn't know much about his life when he was away from them. Justin wasn't getting much guidance about being a teenager. The chaplain and I both tried to help him deal with Minnie's illness and encouraged his involvement with his schoolwork and the sports he loved.

Justin was a delight to them both and he enjoyed their usually upbeat attitude—except for the times Jack had too much to drink. That didn't happen often, but when it did both Minnie and Justin said Jack could be belligerent, loud, and sometimes act in a threatening manner. That was a real problem, and the chaplain and I talked with each member of the family about the drinking.

Jack phoned me one evening. He was very angry. Frustrated, he asked for help, saying maybe Justin couldn't stay with them anymore. Someone had reported to the authorities about Jack's anger, his drinking, and a gun. I talked with him a few minutes on the phone, then talked with Justin, and said I'd be there the next day.

I drove out to see them the following day and spent time with both Jack and Minnie. She said he had been very drunk and had waved a gun around, really frightening them all. Minnie was so angry with him.

"I know he's drinking more because he's worried about me," Minnie said.

He said, "I'd never hurt anyone. But I have to have a gun to protect my family."

"Jack, when you drink, you don't think clearly," I said, trying to help him see the whole picture. "It's dangerous to have a gun in your hand or even in your house then. And it's just unacceptable to have a gun here now."

The compromise for the moment was that Minnie would keep the gun hidden. I picked Justin up from school and took him to a restaurant for burgers and a talk. He told me that he sometimes was afraid of his grandpa.

"I know you love him and you know he loves you. He says he'd never really hurt anyone, just wants to protect his family. Your grandma agrees and says he just needs to yell and look and feel in charge of his family. She's mostly used to it, she says, and he's never hurt anyone." Then I had to ask: "It's important for you to think about this and tell me: Do you feel safe there?"

Justin was quiet a moment, then said, "No."

I could tell it was really hard for him to talk about his fear or say negative things about his grandfather. "No, I don't feel safe when he's like that. The last time he pointed the gun at *me*. I'm afraid of him when he's drinking, even with no gun."

"I'm so sorry, Justin. That's a terrible feeling, and I'm sure it's hard for you to say that. It can't end here. The law requires that I report this. I will talk to the social worker at school and make sure she helps you have protection and counseling. It may be necessary for you to have a foster home—at least for a while. That can be a good thing because there needs to be a solution to where you will live when Minnie passes; maybe this will work out even better than we can imagine now. You could still be with your grandparents when someone is there with you. And our hospice will have to settle the gun issue with them."[4]

Justin seemed relieved, asking, "Can it be a home where there are kids my age?"

There can be difficult decisions when someone is "a danger to themselves or others." Social work guidelines and professional ethics—and the law—require Justin's fear and the danger in the home to be reported. The school social worker did an assessment, worked with the family, found Justin a foster home, and arranged for him to be with his grandparents frequently with supervision. The foster family included students from Justin's school; he moved in with them and became even more involved in school and sports. He seemed to thrive. And he was with his grandparents when it worked out with his foster family and the social worker or when someone from hospice was there. It was in some ways a relief to Jack and Minnie.

Then Jack was diagnosed with terminal lung cancer. What a blow to everyone: Jack, Minnie, Justin, and our team. Soon we were visiting both of them and there were two hospital beds in that narrow living room. We had been caring for Minnie for several months; we would have only several weeks with Jack. They both received the full benefit of hospice: the equipment, medication, and people—nurses, nurse aides, our chaplain, and me.

Just a few weeks later I received a call from the team about Jack's death. It was so difficult for everyone. And what about Minnie now? I thought back over my many visits and my memories with the whole family as I drove to that tiny town, to the mobile home park, and found Justin seated on the front steps, his face buried in his hands. Minnie, inside, was stunned. The nurse was there, and the chaplain arrived soon after. We all cried with them. We comforted them, helped with arrangements for the funeral, and a few days later our chaplain conducted the services. Only a few weeks later, Minnie also died. Her hospice caregivers attended both funerals with Justin. The chaplain and I connected with him after the funeral, and he continued to have good help from the social worker and his foster family. Minnie, Jack, and Justin were very special to our team. There were so many complications and changes for them in a short time. I know the hospice team eased their lives; each one of them enriched our lives.

AL AND JANICE

"I'm not going to shoot anyone."

"Karen, this one's for you," our nurse said in morning staff meeting. "Janice was the one to get out the gun last night. Please go see them soon."

Al, our patient, was in his mid-forties, diagnosed with end-stage cirrhosis of the liver. He spent most of his time in a hospital bed positioned next to a window in the living room of the family's mobile home. A chain smoker and heavy drinker, he was extremely frustrated by his illness and limitations. Janice was busy and exhausted from caring for Al and their four children. No one worked outside their home, and finances were tight. There were six people in the small space, limited money, and multiple frustrations.

Their family included three sons and a tiny sprite of a girl. She had just started school and loved it; the boys, not so much. This delightful little girl had been diagnosed with ADHD and was a live wire. Al explained to me: "I didn't know what that meant, so I asked the doc. He said it's like when you're at Sears watching all the TVs set on the same channel so you can compare them. Except, for her, it's like all the sets are on different channels—so it's really hard for her to concentrate. That must be tough. So I try to understand."

The nurse, the chaplain, and I knew of the family's many difficulties. When the oldest boy got in serious trouble in school and was in the city's juvenile detention for a few days, the chaplain and I visited him there. The other boys were sometimes in detention at school, and I went to talk to them there. At least while they were there they got individual attention and did a little better on their schoolwork with that personal supervision.

The kids built a go-kart with their dad's help. Al gave them directions from his hospital bed guiding them through the screen window. It was good for him to feel a part of some good times in their lives. They loved riding it. The chaplain and I regularly included them in the kids' group.

I already knew about Janice and the gun because Al had called the hospice twenty-four-hour phone number the night before and asked for me to come to their home, saying Janice was acting strange and seemed frantic. He couldn't talk her down. I had gone to the house and found Janice had locked herself in the bathroom with their gun. She opened the door and whispered to me that she had bullets but had not loaded the gun. She let me in and we sat on the bathroom floor as she poured out her frustrations and her worries about Al, the kids, and how depressed she felt.

"I'm not going to shoot anyone. I am so frustrated and sad. Sometimes I just want Al to really listen to me," she said through angry tears." I feel like I'd like to stop all the troubles with Al, his drinking and being so sick and crabby. Sometimes I think about killing myself, but I won't. Who'd do all the work? Who'd take care of the kids?"

"You have so many difficult things going on right now," I said. "The chaplain and I will come more often for a while. Please think about going to one of our support groups, and I'll give you some things to read. We'll arrange for a volunteer to visit with Al while you go out to lunch with me this week. We'll talk more about your discouragement and about the support groups."

"It's very reasonable to be disappointed that your life is so difficult. I want you to think about four Ds—disappointment, discouragement, despair, and depression. Sometimes one follows the other when you don't get enough help. Even depression, as scary as it is, is likely because of the situation you're in. It will likely go away. It doesn't feel like it sometimes, I know. If it continues, we can help you see a therapist and a physician who can help."

"It's so scary . . ." Janice sobbed.

"Yes, I know it is. Andrew Solomon has written a wonderful book about depression. He has written that it was helpful when he determined to manage the discouragement one day at a time, sometimes even one moment at a time, finding that the next moment he was alright, then the next."[5]

We talked a long time. We talked about the multiple problems facing the family. She calmed down and we went out into the living room. She told Al she was sorry; he said, "You scared me, woman!"

Al kept the gun under the mattress of his hospital bed. He said it was so he could protect his family. The next day our chaplain and I talked with them both. Even without bullets ready to be fired, they came to realize that having the gun in the house caused just too much drama and was too hard on the kids, who really had no control over the adult problems or behavior. We couldn't count on Al's good judgment if he did drink. And it was dangerous for anyone who visited; they permitted us to remove the gun from their home.

The chaplain and I, at separate times, talked to both Al and Janice about thoughts of giving up. Both faced bouts of depression. Now that Al wasn't drinking—as far as we knew—he was a bit better physically, but he still was stressed, sad, and discouraged. He was young and his life was so limited. When faced with illness, impending death, financial burdens, and normal, everyday kid issues, both Al and Janice sometimes felt it was too much to handle. With hospice help—medically, spiritually, emotionally, and financially—our patients and family members often learned that they could manage more difficulty than they ever thought possible and still have a relatively good quality of life.

I did not try to have control over Al's smoking, instead learning to pick my battles. However, when he'd light up, I'd say, "Ah, my doctor says I can't breathe that stuff. I'll wait outside 'til you're done."

Now, most of my patients took that statement as a reason to wait to light up until after I left. Not Al; he said, "Oh, honey, I understand. I'll take care of that," and he'd open the window by his bed before he lit up, then he'd take a drag and quickly move the cigarette to the six inches of the open window. Oh, well . . .

After many weeks of good care and no, or very little, drinking, Al actually got better and was discharged from our hospice. Without abuse, a liver may partially regenerate. The healing didn't last long for Al, however. When he didn't feel "terminal," he started drinking. He came back on our hospice program when he became very ill again, continued to decline, and died in a few weeks.

The kids and I created the memorial brochure with Al's favorite hymns and poems that we picked out together. Their hospice nurse visited after the service, and the chaplain and I continued to see the children and Janice for a while. Janice got a job that helped her meet people, get out of the house, and have the money the family needed.

Chapter Seven

Social Isolation

A full and satisfying life is available to most Americans, including a family, home, education, work, leisure activities, personal relationships, freedom, safety, and health care. Isolation from any of these things due to stigmas relating to age, religion, incarceration, LGBTIQ[1] status, mental illness, social class, physical disability, lack of good health care, or a personal inability to maintain quality relationships diminishes individual joy and social cohesion. All of these damage individuals and society as a whole. The three stories in this chapter address three isolated individuals—a female prisoner, an angry man, and an HIV/AIDS patient.

An ideology—a system of beliefs and values—provides our worldview. When that worldview defines one group of persons as superior to another, the consequences are that some folks are highly valued while others are not. For instance, replace the phrase "one group of persons . . ." with "a straight person is superior to a gay person" and the results are that the gay person will be treated unjustly. Hospice treats everyone equally.

Isolation is inherent in many aspects of living and dying with HIV/AIDS, often beginning as soon as parents, siblings, other family members, and even friends learn someone identifies themselves as part of the LGBTIQ community. Thankfully, the opposite is also true, and family and friends often learn to help one another.

Sometimes individuals create their own isolation by living their life in anger.

Prisons vary greatly from town to town, state to state, and even in the federal prison system. In some facilities, prisoners have the benefit of hospice care. The National Hospice Association (NPHA)[2] provides a network of community hospices and correction facilities in an effort to provide good patient care in prison. In some cases, "compassionate release" may be available.

JULIE AND HER MOM

"She's dying of cancer. She's in prison."

Hospice will always be a part of me; the experiences there helped me in my next job as director of patient services in a regional office of the American Cancer Society (ACS). I worked with cancer patients and their families and health care professionals, listening, providing information, creating and monitoring support groups, providing transportation to treatment, and working with other community organizations, including hospice.

One morning as I was working on plans for an ACS volunteer training session with a colleague, Early Detection Director Terese, my assistant called to me from the other room: "Karen, I need you to take this call. It's a mother—her daughter has cancer, and she's in prison . . ."

I picked up the phone: "Hello, this is Karen, how can I help?"

"I don't know what to do. I'm so worried about my daughter . . ."

"Tell me about her." I indicated to Terese that I'd like her to wait while I learned about the situation and gave the caller some information. I thought it would just take a minute or two.

"She's dying. She's in prison in south Texas and she has cancer and. . . . Well, she's dying. That's why suddenly they're releasing her to come home tomorrow. She says they'll only give her enough pain medicine for six hours; it takes longer than that to get here. I just don't know what to do. It's all so terrible . . ." She was weeping.

"Oh, my dear, that's so difficult. I'm glad you called us. I'm sorry she's so sick; it seems wonderful that she can be released, but I can understand your worries. What is her name?"

"Julie."

"First, can Julie live with you when she gets here?"

"Well, I want her to, but I don't know how to take care of her. I don't know how to get her medicine; I can't even afford a doctor for myself. This is going to be so expensive. I just don't know what to do . . ."

"Do you know about hospice care for people who are dying?"

"I've heard of it, but I'm sure I can't afford it."

"Well, here's the first good news for you: Hospice takes care of terminally ill patients in their home and it doesn't cost the patient or the family a thing."

"Really? That is the best news I've had in a long, long time. What do I do? "

"First let *me* do some things. Tell me more about you and Julie, then I'll phone an oncologist I know, a cancer specialist, who works with hospice. I'll call you back in just a few minutes. Please give me your name and phone number . . ."

I wrote down the basic information I needed, hung up, took a deep breath, and said, "Oh, my gosh!"

"Yeah, no kidding," Terese said.

"This woman's daughter has cancer; she's being released from prison tomorrow—she has no meds . . ."

"I think I got most of the story," Terese said as she stood up and headed for the door. "You obviously have some work to do; I'll see you later. You go, girl."

My mind was in a whirl. The thing that stopped me for a bit was just thinking about what that patient in prison and her mom had been through. What flashed through my mind included thoughts about Julie's life leading to prison, being locked up, then being diagnosed with cancer—the emotional and physical pain and the fear of looking ahead. And now the cancer was terminal. For this mother's daughter, now there was cancer pain as well, and a lot of emotional pain, sadness, and feeling out of control.

I phoned the hospice physician I knew best, explained the situation, and asked, "Will you see her?"

"Of course," she said. "Let me know when she gets into town and I'll meet her at my office—any time, day or night. Have her mom request any paperwork she can get from the prison officials—medical history including the cancer diagnosis and any other conditions, a list of medications she's receiving, discharge orders, the name and phone numbers of the doctors who have treated her there, and any other records they'll give her. If things are as the mother described, I'll be able to get her some meds and into hospice ASAP."

I gave the physician the information I had, then phoned Julie's mother and gave her the good news: "It's all set: A really kind and wonderful oncologist is ready to see Julie as soon as she gets into town—anytime tomorrow. She'll examine her and get her the medication she needs right away. The paperwork and the doctor's examination mean she'll most likely get her into hospice right away. Be sure to get as much paperwork from the prison as you can. Write this down, please, I'll go slowly . . ." I gave her the list of information the doctor had requested.

"Now, about hospice. First, the medications will not be a problem; the doctor will order what Julie needs. We'll have the hospice nurse come to your home; she'll meet you and Julie and give you the whole picture. She will do a physical assessment, order the ongoing medication and the medical equipment Julie will need, and give you some guidance."

"A hospice nurse will visit in your home, usually twice a week, and there's a nurse on call for questions or emergencies. They will send a home health aide for a couple of hours a day when Julie needs that kind of help, and there is a chaplain and a social worker who will visit. These folks won't be staying with you all the time—but they are available by phone twenty-four-hours a day and will come to the house when necessary. They will help you know how to care for Julie. None of it costs you or Julie anything."

Her relief was palpable, even over the phone. She wept and said, "I didn't know this was even possible."

"There's more good news: Julie can have any equipment she needs. It's part of the hospice help—the hospital bed, a walker, a wheelchair, whatever, will be delivered to your home. I'll call you in a few days when Julie is settled in to see how things are going, and I'll tell you about the support groups ACS offers, for her and for you. In the meantime, be sure to call me if you have any questions."

"Thank you so much. Oh, thank you!"

Later that morning, Terese and I attended the monthly ACS board meeting. The board was made up of ACS staff and volunteers from the community—physicians, business persons, nurses, social workers, and other community leaders. These professionals provide advice and information, and they help with plans and decisions about ACS programs and services. Volunteers are also on policy-making committees and the boards at the local, state, and national level of ACS. Each month, each department director gives a short report.

I gave my department report, then said, "I have a story for you. This morning I received a phone call from a woman whose daughter is being released from prison *tomorrow*; she has cancer . . ." and I described the story of Julie and her mother's dilemma and how I was able to connect them to a hospice physician who will see Julie and make an assessment as soon as she gets in town, get her the meds she needs, and admit her to hospice. "And I told her about our ACS support groups and Road to Recovery volunteers."

It was a joy to give those community leaders a better understanding of the work of my department through a story of a real family currently in crisis. Terese leaned over and whispered to me, "Now I understand why a social worker is needed in your job."

DON

"There's nothing you can do for me."

I made my first visit to my patient Don early one evening; I remember it being dark outside when I arrived, and his wife Louise greeted me at the door. Inside, I felt a hushed sadness; more than that, there was a heaviness in the house. It felt "dark" inside too. Don's family members greeted me, keeping their voices low. They motioned to an open door off the living room where I could see the end of a double bed, indicating Don's room, then invited me to sit with them before I saw Don. I knew he was bedfast and very ill.

In a very quiet voice, Louise introduced me to the family that filled the small living room: an adult daughter and a son-in-law, their son and his wife, and a middle-aged cousin, Tom. Any talking was done quietly; it seemed they wanted to keep anything happening between them away from the patient. Don was only fifty-seven; I'm sorry to say that I don't even remember his diagnosis. What I remember is the ambiance of that house.

"You can go in there, but he won't talk much," Louise said. "He does want to know who's here, so go ahead in when you want to. Tom will go with you when you're ready. He's about the only one Don talks to now."

"Thanks, I'll go in to see him in a few minutes. I'd like to learn a bit about you and see how I can help," I said, sitting down. Most of the folk sat then, and when they interacted with me it was done in a subdued manner.

"I'm so sorry this is happening to Don and to you folks. It's very hard to be so sick and hard to know how to help sometimes. What do you find helps him the most?"

"Well, it sure isn't talking about any of this." Don's son said.

"We just learned about this a week ago," one of daughters offered.

Don's son-in-law said, "Mostly he's mad. He's mad all the time."

"People have so many reactions to being really sick," the "social worker words" came out of my mouth. "Anger and fear go together, especially when they know they are not going to get better. And it's all so new to you." True, but it still seemed so inadequate.

Don's wife Louise said, "Of course, that's kinda how he is, mad. He gets mad real easy, stays mad mostly, and he doesn't like to talk much."

Louise's daughter said quietly, "I can't remember when he wasn't mad. And he never wants to talk much about anything. It's always been like that."

From the bedroom came an angry voice: "Who is that? They comin' in here or not?"

"It's the social worker from hospice," Louise said to him from the living room.

"Good grief!"

Tom motioned for me to follow him into the bedroom; the door was wide open, and there was no privacy from the folks gathered in the living room. Louise said quietly, "You go ahead. I'll make some coffee."

There was no place to sit in the tiny bedroom. *No problem*, I thought, *I likely won't be in here long.* Tom went to stand by the opposite side of the bed, and I said, "Hi, Don, I'm Karen. I'm from hospice. I understand you've felt bad quite a while and just found out what's wrong. You didn't get very good news. I'm sorry you're having to deal with this; it's hard to be sick."

"You wouldn't be here if I was well, right? Had lots of folk comin' by. Don't see any of 'em really helpin' except that nurse. Them pills helps a lot."

"So you are more comfortable now with the medications, that's good. Tell her if there's anything else—nausea, anything. Is there anything else you need?"

"Yeah, I need a new body."

"It's good your family lives nearby and can be here. I'm guessing that helps—it sure helps your wife to have them here. I'll talk to you about anything you'd like . . ."

"Nope."

"I'll spend some time with your family, maybe that's the best way I can help."

"Up to them . . ." He didn't make eye contact, didn't really want to talk more.

"If you change your mind, they can call me, and I'll come back when you like."

"There's nothin' you can do for me."

Wisely, Tom stayed with Don, and I walked back out into the living room. Louise motioned for me to go into the kitchen with her. We sat at the small kitchen table and talked a bit about how *she* was and who was helping her. The message I got verbally, and from the behavior of everyone in that house, was that Don was an angry, sullen, mostly quiet man. When he spoke, the words and the tone were often ugly. Hospice team members had already told me about his anger and negativity.

Louise said, "I don't remember the last time he said anything nice to me."

"It's very hard to live with negativity; I'm so glad you have family nearby. You and I can talk now if you like, and if and when it's reasonable, I'd love to go to lunch with you, maybe in a day or two; we can go when the home health aide is here for a couple of hours, and we can really talk," I said. "You have all been having a really rough time. And it's all so new—the diagnosis, hospice, the medical equipment, the visitors . . ."

"Yes, it's really hard. But he's never nice, mostly been angry—for a long, long time. He only agreed to go to the doctor when he got to hurting so bad. It's wonderful the pain is better; that helps a lot. It helps him—it also helps us. He sleeps better now."

We talked a few minutes, then her daughter joined us. "It's hard to try to be close, it's hard to help. He's always been cross most of the time, and now it's worse."

"Don's anger reminds me of an ancient quote from Seneca the Younger: 'Anger is an acid that can do more harm to the vessel in which it is stored than to anything on which it is poured.'[3] It's hard on you and it's been hard on him. I'm sorry you and he have had to deal with this for so long. It makes saying goodbye difficult and also it may be a relief. Let's get together again soon."

I learned the next day that Don had died early in the morning. I phoned Louise, my heart going out to that family. I told her I'd go to the funeral and see them there, and then I'd visit her again in a few days. Now my heart went out to our chaplain, Marty, who had been asked to do the service. What could he say?

The service was in the church Louise and the kids attended. They were well known there. It was a large church, and there were over a hundred people in attendance, many folks stopping by with hugs and kind words for Louise and the kids as they sat in the front row. We listened to the organ music, and I kept thinking about our chaplain and praying for his wisdom. I wondered what Don's life had been like, what sadness there was that made him so bitter and angry. Whatever has happened in a person's life, there are positive things that can be said about most folks. The hospice team members who had cared for Don all said that they never heard a kind word from him or about him.

The organ music stopped and the church pastor, a friend of the family, and our chaplain walked onto the platform. The pastor prayed (I was told he did not know Don), and the friend read the obituary. Then our chaplain went to the pulpit. The floor of the platform was about three feet above the casket, and to make things even more difficult, the casket was open.

Many people in the church were there to support the family; they didn't know Don well. Those who knew him had likely experienced his sullenness and anger. Marty, who had visited Don recently, now talked about the love of God for all persons, about how He had even shared his own Son with human-ity. He spoke candidly about Don having difficulties, anger, and negative feelings. I could see people exchanging glances, nodding their agreement. Marty talked about Jesus as kind spoken and tender hearted, knowing our experiences, our frustrations, and fears, sadness, and anger.

And he said, "If Jesus were here right now, what would he say?"

Then Marty stretched his arm over the top of the pulpit, down toward where Don's body was lying in that open casket, and said, "I believe he would reach down his hand just like I am doing now and he would say: 'Don, I love you, I understand you; I know about the hard things in your life, and I know your sad and angry feelings. I love you. You are mine. I offer you the peace you didn't seem to have during most of your life on this earth. I want you to have peace . . .'"

There was more, but that is what has stayed in my mind and heart. He concluded with: "Don and I hold hands today in spirit as I pray for him . . ." It was truly redemptive, beautiful, and healing for the family and for me.

Don had said there was nothing we could do for him; we helped manage his symptoms and we were there for his family during his final days and after his death.

BRYCE AND HIS DAD

The social deaths and psychological pain of AIDS patients.

Early one afternoon, I parked in front of a lovely home in a quiet neighborhood. The yard was filled with beautiful trees, and I enjoyed the earthy smell of fresh mulch in the neat beds of flowers and shrubs in the well-manicured lawn. That ambiance helped me feel peaceful and calm as I prepared emotionally for this visit. Inside, our patient Bryce was near the end of his battle with AIDS.[4] He was living with his father, Ed, now his caregiver. Our intake nurse had shared with me that they hadn't been close for years.

Ed invited me in, and I asked if we could sit and talk before I saw his son. Sitting in the lovely brown leather chairs, the sunlight filtering in through the windows touching the wood and leather, and I felt I was in a safe, warm place. I shared that feeling with Ed: "This lovely, peaceful environment must be really helpful to Bryce."

"I hope so. I felt like my son was already dead to me when I learned he was gay—now this. I really don't know how to manage."

Ed wanted to talk, needed to: "Years before, when I learned that Bryce was gay, I told him I didn't want to be around him or his friends. It was the mid-1980s, we'd heard about 'those people' who were spreading a frightening new disease. I'm sorry to say that I told Bryce I wasn't surprised that he and his friends were reaping what they had sown with their unacceptable choices. I couldn't accept that Bryce was one of them, and I told him I would not see him again."

"I'm so ashamed now that I couldn't accept him, stay close to him—even if I didn't like his choices. Now people tell me that being that way isn't something people choose; I just don't know. I do love him and want to help him."

"Thank you for sharing those painful thoughts," I said quietly. "You are doing a wonderful thing now—welcoming him here, trying to understand, learning how to help. Now perhaps you can be close again."

Ed said they were trying to be comfortable with each other, talking again about their history and their family and finding the good things they still shared as father and son. Both were working to accept this new normal.

"Ed, dealing with HIV/AIDS has been difficult for everyone—for patients, families, and caregivers," I said. "We still have so much to learn about it and about how to care for these patients. Have you read about the HIV virus? The nurse can give you medical information; I'd like to talk to you about your other questions. Tell me about Bryce and your family . . ."

Ed shared some of their histories. He said Bryce had been a good student. He liked music rather than sports. "I tried to help him with the sports stuff he needed to know, you know, throwing softballs, catching footballs. . . . His mother and I were so surprised and sad to learn he was gay. I just couldn't handle it; that's not the only reason, but our pain and the disagreements are part of the reason the wife and I divorced a few years ago." It was obvious both Bryce and Ed had experienced much loneliness and sadness through all the changes.

"Tell me about Bryce coming here, coming home."

"He's so sick. It was hard for him to tell me . . . anything. But I know his friends, his boyfriend, couldn't care for him anymore."

"This is a good thing you've done, having him here with you. A good thing for him and for you. How's it going?"

"You know, it's so much easier than I thought it would be. It's good to talk to him, and I'm trying to understand and accept what I don't understand. It's been hard to believe he's going to die from this AIDS thing. The hospice nurses are a huge help to both of us—they help me understand what's going on physically and show me how I can help."

"What a blessing for you both," I said. "Now you understand how HIV/AIDS patients have two deaths—a social death and the psychological pain it causes, and the physical illness and death. They deal with multiple physical problems, fatigue, and often this particular skin cancer Bryce has now, and sometimes a special type of pneumonia. And they live with the likelihood that they'll die much younger than they'd imagined. You are now experiencing all that with him. Is there anything else you'd like to talk about right now? I will be back in a week or so. And you can call me to come anytime"

"No, go in to see him. Maybe next time we can talk some more. Oh, wait, I do have a worry. I cry so easily. I don't want to make things harder on him."

"Does it seem to bother him?'

"He says, 'Dad, it's okay. I cry too, I just love being here with you.'"

"I think you've done the very best thing you can do for him, having him here with you. The tears are healthy; they are acknowledging all kinds of things: the difficult past, seeing him so ill, the frustration of learning what to do now, and knowing that he will die. They show him how much you love him, and he knows you'll understand his crying and sadness. And likely tears are a relief . . ."

"That's true. Thanks. Okay, I'll take you to Bryce's room."

The door was open and Ed introduced me to Bryce, then left. I greeted Bryce and sat on a chair near his bed. He was very ill. The blue and purple blotches of Kaposi sarcoma, "the AIDS cancer," were evident, especially on his arms. There were some on his face. He was very thin, and he seemed very tired. The hospice team was concerned and watching for evidence of the pneumocystis pneumonia that also often afflicts AIDS patients' lungs.

"I'm so very happy to have you folks—hospice helps me so much, and it helps my Dad. That's really important—this is so hard on him," Bryce said.

We had a good talk and he described how helpful it was to have this new, more open relationship with his dad: "Dad's alone; I'd thought that one day he'd accept me. I thought when he was old and needed me, I could help him. Now it's the other way around."

"It's wonderful that he's opening up to you and helping—it's good for him too, you know. How do you spend your time with him?"

"We watch old movies and that brings up things he'll talk about, things important to him, things I didn't know about his past. I'm learning so much about him. That part is really good."

Then I asked Bryce, "Tell me about your partner if you're comfortable with that."

"I miss him. But I understand and it's fine. I love him; it's hard to be apart. We were partners for nine years, we owned our own home together. After a while it just got too hard—he couldn't keep his job and take care of me. I haven't worked in a long time. I had a good job, had health insurance, had life insurance. None of it anymore. None. You know those companies who buy your life insurance and give you cash?[5] Well, I did that. I don't know if it was the best thing, but I had the money to stay there for a while, then it helped with the move here, and I can help dad a bit with expenses. That money is mostly gone—there's just enough for a funeral."

"It's okay. It is what it is. I made choices and here I am. It's pretty much me and my dad now. He and I are trying to understand each other. It's good to be here—but it's not my own home. I miss my lover and my friends. Dad says it's good I'm here and tries to understand. The time passes slowly . . ."

"Let your dad do things for you. He feels so helpless—let him borrow films, books, or books on tape for you from the library, buy you magazines, special foods you like and can tolerate. You might even watch *And the Band Played On*[6] with him. That might give him helpful background info and bring out some answers for him, and he may ask you questions he's not been able to ask so far."

"Aren't you afraid?" Bryce asked me. "Everyone else is . . . afraid of being with me, touching me."

"No, I'm not—we're not. All of us at hospice have been learning about HIV/AIDS, we attend workshops to learn more. Also, now our staff actually gives workshops in the community about it. We know it's only spread by sharing fluids—and if we do some procedure where that's possible, we wear gloves. And you understand that too, I think. I hope you know that our wearing gloves doesn't have anything to do with you as a person. We wear gloves when we're helping patients with many kinds of illnesses. You have a compromised immune system—the precaution of gloves is to protect you from getting something from us as well."

"Thanks for that . . ."

"Scientists are working hard on understanding HIV/AIDS; there will be more help one day soon. Each of us is here for you and your dad. Do you have anything special you'd like to talk about right now?"

"I've made a really good connection with the chaplain and we talk a lot," Bryce said. "I appreciate you, but please help my dad."

"Yes, we will, however we can. There are community support groups I'll tell him about—HIV/AIDS support groups are as much about sharing information as giving support. It's almost always helpful to hear others' stories and be able to ask honest questions, express frustrations, and learn about caretaking. I'll urge him to go to one of those."

"Thanks," Bryce said softly. "It's all so hard."

"Take care—see you soon, in about two weeks likely. Please call if you'd like me to come sooner—for you or your dad."

Bryce died with his dad at his bedside, holding his hand, a few weeks later.

Chapter Eight

Saying Goodbye

It was a precious part of my job and an honor for me to find ways to help folks say goodbye to partners, spouses, parents, grandchildren, children, siblings, and friends, even in complicated family situations, managing multiple losses, fear, anger, great love, or cultural differences.

Many things may contribute to a person's concerns about dying: They may wonder "What's it like to die?" "What is next?" "How will my family cope?" They may be afraid of losing control or may want to make things right with someone. Hospice personnel are especially attuned to the emotional and spiritual needs of patients, listening carefully, open to talking freely about anything, and supporting the strengths they receive from their belief system.

When possible, we helped patients participate in the practices important to them at the end of life—last rites, laying on of hands, or some other personal rite of passage. Death doulas[1] are available also, spending quality time with families, assisting with death as birth doulas assist with births.

One lovely ritual is called "holding space." It's offering time, in a non-judgmental, accepting way, a "withness" as people transition into death. The concept is described beautifully by Heather Plett,[2] writer, coach, and facilitator, writing of the death of her mother and the help from her palliative care nurse. There are many other circumstances and ways this concept of "being with" can be used. In this first story, you'll learn that Frank and Viola were welcomed into the family room of their children as Viola became more fragile and her death was near in order for family to surround her much of the day and night.

Chapter 8

FRANK AND VIOLA

"What's happening next week, honey?"

I first met Frank and Viola in their daughter's home. She and her family invited them to move in with them during Viola's final illness. Her hospital bed was placed in one corner of their great room—the kitchen, dining room, and media area. That thoughtful arrangement meant Viola could enjoy watching the busy family life continuing around her. Frank helped the teens with homework, washed the dishes, and slept on the hide-a-bed near her, watching TV late into the night. The lights and sounds near Viola were kept low; she slept much of the time now.

The hospice nurses and I talked with the whole family, helping them understand some of the changes they could expect: increased fatigue, sleeping more, loss of appetite, breathing changes, hands and feet feeling cool to the touch as her body began shutting down and circulation diminished, and feeling a bit confused sometimes. We encourage them to place family photo albums near her bed where the family could look at them with Viola and Frank and talk about special times together. The family took pictures of some of those "being with" times.

Viola, Frank, and I were talking about how they met, their life together, and their children and grandchildren when Frank said, "Honey, what's happening next week?"

"Our anniversary," Viola said, smiling at him fondly.

She was pleasant and calm. She wasn't hungry and hadn't eaten for days. The family asked if we needed to give her a feeding tube, and we described to them that artificial nutrition and hydration would likely make her physically uncomfortable because her body just couldn't process food easily anymore. Too much nutrition could overburden her system and might cause swelling in her abdomen or legs. We explained that she was in the process of dying, and this shutting down was to be expected. Still, it was difficult for the family—caregiving seemed to them to mean preparing food and urging her to eat and drink.

That first day I visited, Viola said she wasn't thirsty either and really didn't want to drink anything. It was hard for the family to believe she didn't at least need some water. We supplied them with medicated swabs to moisten her lips. Much of the time she kept her eyes closed, resting, listening, or sleeping.

Family activities continued nearby—meals were cooked and eaten where she could watch, the grandchildren sat at the edge of her bed now and then, and friends were coming and going. She would talk to them for just a few moments, then rest again. They were all rethinking what caring for her meant. They wanted to give her the best care possible; now they were learning to shift their definition of care.

Every person has the right to refuse treatment. It's in the First Amendment.[3] That includes food and water. It's good to know that, but it's different from seeing someone you love making those choices. On the wall near Viola's bed was a "Do Not Resuscitate" (DNR) sign.[4] Medical folks know that the resuscitation of a frail, elderly person often results in lots of trauma to his or her body.[5] It was important that the family understood all these possibilities and that they came to support the decision Viola had made—no more heroic treatment of any kind.

"Call us at hospice, don't call 911. She doesn't want that kind of help," I reminded them. And if someone panics and calls 911, the EMTs and paramedics are mandated to work to resuscitate her. You need to point out the DNR to the medical technicians. That allows them to not try to resuscitate her.

My second visit with Frank and Viola was just a few days later in the hospital. Their daughter wanted to care for her at home, then she and her husband became concerned that perhaps grandma dying in their home would be too hard on the kids and asked our hospice for other options. We arranged for a room in the nearby hospital where only comfort care would be given.

The family came to visit often, taking turns so someone was there with her much of the time. This arrangement was just more comfortable for them, and Viola and Frank understood. Some hospices have their own hospice house for this type of care. When Frank or the family was with Viola, they still tried to get her to sip water. It's very hard to do nothing and they often moistened her lips with the swabs. Just being with her was everything at that point. She was so calm, peaceful, and untroubled—and not hungry, thirsty, or in pain.

During this visit alone with Viola, she and I talked about how she felt physically and emotionally and I asked what she might need or want. She said she was comfortable and at peace. Then Frank came into the room: "Honey, what's happening next week?"

And she answered, as always, with a smile: "Our anniversary."

The three of us talked and I asked them to tell me more about special times in their lives. When I left, Frank followed me out into the hall. He asked if we could just sit together for a few minutes. He talked about his sadness and his concerns; he said he knew we were doing our best and knew she couldn't live long.

Then he said, "How long do you think it will be? How long can she do it?"

"How long can she do what?" I asked.

"How can she keep going, keep living? No food; almost no water. She seems to be comfortable, but how can she keep living?"

"Frank," I said, "Each person's journey is their own—medically and emotionally. She still enjoys seeing you and the rest of the family. And she's calm and seems very comfortable. The time will come. What do you ask her every time you see her?"

"I don't know. I talk about the kids; I tell her I love her. What?"

"Frank, think a minute—what did you ask her when you came into the room today?"

He thought for just a moment. Then, startled, he said, "No, it can't be! Is she waiting for our anniversary?"

"I don't know. It's not the first time someone waited for someone or something. It's okay, Frank. She loves having you ask that, reminding her of how long you've been married. She enjoys having you tell her you love her. She's okay. It's her timing, not yours. Don't worry about it now, and after the anniversary tell her it's okay if she's too tired and wants to go. Tell her you'll miss her and you'll understand and be okay."

He was incredulous. He said he'd have to think more about that, and he would try to do that for her. He'd continue to celebrate their love, have every moment he could with her, and get ready to let her go. Very soon after their anniversary, she died quietly with her family around her, a hospice nurse attending, and Frank holding her hand.

CINDY AND TIMMY

"It's time to say 'goodbye.'"

"Can you come? Right now, tonight . . . ? The kids would like you to come." Judy, our patient's daughter, asked our hospice operator to have me phone her. She spoke quietly and slowly into the phone: "The nurse says Dad doesn't have much time left. Can you come?" she asked again, "Right now, and help the little ones?"

"Absolutely. I'm so glad you called. I'll be there in a few minutes."

Cindy and Timmy, aged seven and nine, were temporarily living in their grandparents' home. They and their mom had moved there a few weeks before so they all could help with their grandpa's care. The kids were wonderful—helping their mom and grandma in whatever needed doing. Our nurse had talked with them about what was happening physically to their grandpa, and I'd described to them about how hospice was helping and what to expect as he got weaker. The chaplain and I had listened to them at various times, talked to them about their fears, and answered their questions. I had focused on their memories with him and what they could do right now to help. They were really sweet kids, watching and learning how families care for each other.

When I arrived at their home that last evening, the hospice nurse was already there. We all hugged (hospice folks are great huggers) and greeted everyone. I talked with the adults a bit and they went into grandpa's room. Then I sat on the living room sofa with Cindy and Timmy. They said they knew he'd gotten even sicker, but they were afraid and didn't know what to do or say. "His eyes stay closed . . ."

"The good thing is that he's comfortable, he is not hurting," I told them. "He's probably hearing some of what's happening part of the time; other times he's sleeping very deeply. The best thing you can do for him right now is to quietly be with him. Let's plan what to do. We'll go in and you can sit on the bed, put your hand on his arm, tell him your name, and that you're going to be with him. You can talk to him and tell him what you remember about special things—his stories, places he took you. Tell me some of the places you remember . . ."

They remembered times at the zoo, the park, the mall, and fishing.

Cindy asked, "Will he feel bad if I talk about fishing? He loved fishing. He taught us how. We went so many times. Will it make him sad if we talk about it?"

"I think he'll be so happy to remember, too, and to know how much fun it was for you. You could say something like: 'When we go fishing, we'll always think of you. You taught us how to do it right.'" I could see them gaining courage to go be with him.

"Even though he's too sick to talk much, he may be able to hear you, and it will feel good to him to hear your voices. He'll love knowing you remember his stories and the things you've done together. Remember last week when you read one of your favorite books to him? He heard you then and talked about things in the book, and he loved that. You can read another book to him if you like. We'll see if there's time for that."

"Grandma has been in there a lot. She cries when she comes out . . ."

"I know, it's hard for her and for everybody to see him like he is now, to know he's not going to get better. It's okay if you cry in there—it lets him know how much you love him. And tell him you love him. Are you ready? Let's go in together. You let me know when you're comfortable and I'll go out if you like, or I'll stay. You let me know. And each of you can have time with him by yourself with him, to say just what you want to in private if you like. It's time to say 'goodbye.'"

Both kids went in with me, we sat on the bed, and they laid their hands on his arm. And they talked to him. Soon Cindy was ready to talk to him alone; we all left so she could do that. When she came out of the room, Timmy asked me to go in with him while he talked to his grandpa. The adults each had their moments alone with him, then we all sat with him while he took his last quiet breaths. The sad tears were mixed with the joy of new memories made together, helping him.

I knew those kids would have wonderful memories of helping. It was good for them, helping their grandpa, and it was wonderful that they helped their grandma and their own mom and were able to be part of the care themselves. The kids learned the value of helping and of remembering and talking about tough things. And they created new really important memories for themselves.

It is good for each family member to have the opportunity to talk alone with the dying patient, to be able to say anything about anything—sharing good memories or asking for or giving forgiveness. Saying those things can be healing and are helpful to a son or daughter, partner, parent, or friend. It certainly was helpful to me. When my father was comatose after his last stroke, I talked to him about my mom, thanking him again for caring for her through her illnesses. I thanked him for special things he'd made possible for me. We had those private moments together. Each family member took that special time. Then, together, we stood around his bed; he was on life support, but we were honoring his wishes to not have that kind of care. The respirator was removed, and in a few moments, he died quietly with people who loved him talking to him and touching him. It was as good as it could be under the circumstances.

Bereavement counselor Kate Sutton writes a blog about talking with children about death. She offers excellent guidelines using a clever memory device focusing on TALK—important to be truthful, to acknowledge feelings, to listen, and to keep routines consistent.[6]

JIM AND SHARI

"His, hers, ours, and theirs . . ."

"His, hers, ours, and theirs" is how Jim and Shari described their family. They each had a child from a previous relationship, then they married and had a child together. Many folks are part of a family like that.

Jim and Shari loved the idea of their blended family of five, which eventually included two more children. Shari explained, "Jim's brother and his wife died in a terrible auto accident. They had two children and we adopted them. So 'theirs' are now 'ours.' And now we have five children—his, hers, ours, and theirs. The kids love giving that description to their friends!"

Each family is unique. The chaplain and I did our best to interact with Jim, each child, and Shari during Jim's illness and afterward. To do that well takes time. By my second visit, Jim had gotten much worse. It's very difficult to be thorough if the patient is not on our service very long. I was just beginning to get to know the family.

"Karen, let's talk with the kids just a few minutes," Shari said when she met me at the door of their home. "Then I'd like you to come with me to see Jim by ourselves; we can talk to the kids again after."

"Sure, that sounds like a good plan," I said, and we went into the living room and sat with the kids. "How are things, kiddos? Tell me about the time you've spent with your dad this week . . ."

Several of the children shared things they'd done with and said to their dad. Then I asked, "Have each of you had some time alone with him, just talking about what you wanted to by yourself with him?" Most of them had.

The littlest girl said, "Daddy doesn't talk much anymore."

"Ah, but I'll bet he loves to hear your voice," I said. "And he likes to hear your stories about your school and friends. You can even sing to him, or read one of the books you like very much."

One of the children asked, "Is it still okay for me to crawl on the bed with him?"

"If he says it's okay—and check with your mom."

"Can he still hear me when he's got his eyes closed?"

"We believe he can, and I think even the sounds of your voices can make him feel better, and warm and safe. We don't know for sure how much he hears or understands right now."

The oldest boy talked about how much his Dad had changed in just a few days, saying they were frightened by the sounds he made breathing."

"I understand," I said. "As he gets sicker it's harder for him to breathe; the sounds are because of that, kinda like a rattle, right? Sometimes he may even seem to stop breathing for a short time; that kind of breathing even has a special name. It's called Cheyne-Stokes breathing. If he does that, just sit quietly, put your hand on his arm, and tell him you're there with him. There may be a long time between breaths. It can be scary, but it's normal for how sick he is. I'm so proud of all of you. Your mom has told me you have been reading the book for kids about hospice patients that I brought last time; good for you! You want to understand what's happening, don't you? It's not quite so scary when you know that what's happening. This is what we expect when he is so sick."

They knew he would not get better. "He likely hears what you say, even though he doesn't talk to you. It's good to ask questions and talk *about* him out here, then talk *to* him when you're in there. You're all doing such a good job. I'm going to go in to see him with your mom for a few minutes, okay?"

"Good job, Shari," I said, putting my arm around her waist as we walked into the room. "You're really helping the kids by keeping them involved, encouraging them to talk to you, to him, and to us."

Just before we went into the room, Shari confided very quietly: "I'm really afraid; I don't know what to do. He's not eating at all, and not drinking much water. I'm using those swabs to moisten his lips. He sleeps most of the time now. And sometimes he does that funny breathing like you said, where he takes a breath and then doesn't take one for a really long time. But he doesn't move around like he's hurting or anything."

"Yes, that kind of breathing is because his disease is affecting the respiratory system; it's a normal part of the dying process," I explained.

"And his hands and feet feel cold. I've been reading that information the nurse gave me about the signs he's dying. I think maybe he is dying right now."

"When the circulation slows down, his hands and feet will feel cold to us, but likely he doesn't notice it; it's okay."

We went into the room and Jim seemed to be sleeping. Moving closer, Shari sat on the edge of the bed and put her hand on his arm. "Honey, it's me, Shari. Karen's here, can you say 'Hi'?"

He opened his eyes for just a few seconds, murmured something I couldn't understand, and closed his eyes again. His breathing was very shallow and slow.

"He's really tired. He sleeps most of the time."

"That's alright, Jim." I touched his hand gently, then sat on a chair next to the bed. "Your body is really tired; it just isn't letting you talk much right now. You rest; we're going to sit here with you. Shari's going to tell me some special memories of your times together and with your wonderful kids—you just keep resting."

Shari talked, keeping her hand on his arm. His breathing changed, slowed even more. She kept talking, reminding him of special memories, telling him she loved him. Then his breathing stopped. She looked at me, frightened, tears rolling down her face. I took her hand. In a few seconds his breathing began again, then stopped again for several seconds, then an intake of air, and his breathing began again.

"See, that's what he's been doing a lot the last couple of hours before you came," she whispered. "I feel like I should call the kids, but I don't want to. I've been thinking I want to do this alone."

"They've had time with him recently. It's your choice. Do you want me to leave?"

"Oh, no. Please stay with me."

"Okay, keep touching him and talk to him if you want. Get on the bed if you want, lie down with him if you like. Tell him whatever you want."

She quietly told him she loved him, told him again. "We'll be okay, Jim," she said. Then quietly he stopped breathing. This time he didn't breathe again.

Tears came to us both. Quiet tears. Shari sat there with him, motionless, for a few minutes. Then she hugged him and told him she loved him. We sat just a few minutes more, and then she told me she was ready to go tell the children. She wanted me with her when she told them.

We sat with the children and Shari said, "Daddy's gone, he died just now." They cried, of course, and one little one climbed onto Shari's lap. "He wasn't hurting . . ."

We talked a bit more, then I phoned hospice. The chaplain and nurse were soon on their way. We sat together, quiet at first, then Shari talked about Jim, reminding the kids of special things in their lives. We told the kids we'd take them in to see Jim when they were ready.

MR. SANTOS

"We want his body here with us for a while longer."

When I saw the family name of my new patient, Santos, I thought of a friend our family had when we lived in the Republic of the Philippines. I hoped that my knowing a bit of this new family's home country, culture, and a very small amount of Tagalog, the main dialect, might be helpful as we helped them. Mr. Santos had recently chosen to move from active treatment to cure his pancreatic cancer to comfort care in our hospice program.

I was planning to call for an appointment for my first visit when I learned in team meeting that Mr. Santos had already passed. I told the staff I was going anyway, as soon as the family would see me. When I phoned for an appointment, and when a young woman answered, I said, "*Magandang uma-ga, po* [Good morning, with respect]," I began. "This is Karen, the hospice social worker. I'd like to visit your family."

"Yes, ma'am.[7] Oh, my, you know our language. This is Cassie, Mr. Santos's daughter. I am sorry, my father passed a'ready."

"Yes, I know, I'm so sad for your family. Still, I'd like to come meet you and see how I can help."

"Yes, come," she said. And I was not surprised when she explained: "There are many others here, and that's good. You come meet the family, and you can see Mr. Santos too, and sit with us. We want his body here with us for a while longer . . ."

Quickly I relayed that request to the hospice staff; they had not been asked that before. They discussed how long it would be appropriate for Mr. Santos to remain at home. I shared a bit of Filipino culture, especially some customs surrounding death rituals. The team agreed they would give the family a few days for their traditional grieving and sitting with the body, and also to accommodate our American mortuary requirements.

When I arrived at the Santos home, Cassie and an older woman answered the door together. They each put out both hands to take my hands in theirs, tears gleaming through the big smile on each face.

"*Magandang, hapon, po* [Good afternoon, with respect]." I directed this especially to Mrs. Santos. Keeping hold of my hands, they both pulled me into the small living room now filled with people, including small children. Off to the side was a table filled with food: rice and a viand (a mixture of vegetables and meat), fish, lumpia, pancit, oranges, apples, artfully sliced pineapple, and—was it possible?—*calamansi* juice. I couldn't help it; I said to all of them: "I love *calamunsi* juice, and I haven't had any in over ten years!" *Calamansi* is a small round fruit—bright green outside, orange inside, tart and sweeter than a lemon. Lovely as a drink or squeezed into the open end of a *lumpia*.

"*Magandang hapon* [Good afternoon]," I said to all of them and was greeted with happy laughter. They, of course, thought I really knew Tagalog, and began speaking quickly in this common dialect of the Philippines. *That's the danger of a little knowledge*, I thought, and quickly explained: "*Konti, lang* [Just a little]."

I knew I'd be offered some of that wonderful food, but first . . .

"*Pakiusap, ma'am* [Please, madam]," they said, "You come now to see Mr. Santos."

Yes, I was prepared to do that, and prepared to touch him and rub his arm as they did. They had washed and prepared his body and dressed him in his best. He was lying on a single bed in the corner of the living room. His feet were facing the door so that his spirit could depart easily. Mrs. Santos sat down on a chair beside his bed to be as near him as long as possible and to greet the visitors and receive any contributions given. She and many of the others were wearing black; white is allowed, but colorful clothing is discouraged, especially red.

After a few moments, Cassie led me to the table and offered a plate that I filled with the wonderful food; then I sat with the others who were in chairs lining the edges of the small living room. Most of the folk changed from Tagalog to English when I asked about Mr. Santos. They told me many things about his life and his work and his journey to America. They explained that, at home in the Philippines, his body would stay in the home for three days, sometimes up to seven to nine days. I told them I had described some of Filipino traditions to our staff and that hospice would let them keep Mr. Santos with them as long as possible. I said the nurse would call soon to talk about that. There was a mixture of sadness, mourning, and some weeping; still, there was joy because they were together, and family ties were being strengthened as they talked about their memories.

"There will be no sweeping today . . ." I said. (If there is sweeping, it is believed other deaths may follow, and some believe the sweeping pushes good spirits out the door.) There were smiles and an appreciation that I knew that about their culture. "You know, I have many Filipino brooms in my home—I brought them back and I love to use them. They work very well.

Where do you buy them here?" I truly wanted to know a local place where I could replace mine.

In very traditional Filipino families there often are celebrations after the funeral—at least a nine-day "Novena" (prescribed group prayers); another on the fortieth day after the death, said to be the day the person's spirit ascends to heaven; and another celebration is held exactly one year after the death. After that, close family members may again wear colorful clothing. Some do not celebrate birthdays, anniversaries, or other social activities during that first year after a death. This pattern of grieving allows expression of strong grief surrounding the death and encourages accommodation to the grief as the events unfold. Then, when the year of intense mourning is over, it's often easier to move on.

Hospice staff members are fortunate now that they can use the Internet to learn traditional practices surrounding illness and death for the belief system they encounter, and help is also available translating words foreign to them into English. I was happy I had experience with the Filipino culture and could help this grieving family, honoring without violating their customs.

MR. EDWARDS, WOODY ALLEN, AND JANICE

Being there—or not.

A one-story, tastefully painted stucco building stretched along a side street in a small Texas town. Many lovely oak trees arched over the roofline. Walking through the front door of a pleasant skilled nursing facility, I headed for my first meeting with a new patient. Mr. Edwards wanted us to meet not in his room, but in the bright and cheery day room. Tables and chairs were available for games, crafts, puzzles, and snacks, helping make it a pleasant and inviting place. Along the side was a counter with a coffee pot, Texas sweet tea in a jug, hot water for hot tea, boxes full of assorted tea bags, snacks, sodas, and an ice machine. Two residents were chatting and nibbling on snacks a few tables away. The activity room door opened onto a backyard, the inside "U" of the building, and it was filled with trees, flowers, and sunshine. A very pleasant, inviting, open area.

"Hi, Mr. Edwards. I'm Karen, the social worker from hospice. I'm glad you wanted to meet here, it's very nice. Nice inside and out—would you like to sit outside?"

"Good morning. No, let's sit here. Thanks for visiting."

"I'm happy to meet you. How are things? How are you feeling today?"

"Oh, I'm okay. Doing pretty good for how bad they say I am," he said with a grin. "Those nurses have me feeling so much better. Pain's gone; they've got me on some other new meds, too, for stomach problems an' all."

"You just moved here, right? I'm wondering how things are for you here. Do you have any questions or concerns?"

"Nope; it's better than I thought it would be. I've been here a few weeks, and I'm pretty well settled in. I just got the *really* bad news. Cancer, I didn't know 'til just a few days ago. I'm getting lots of attention now. Nice you folks are coming too. I guess the nurses from hospice help the nurses here. My friends here are going to get jealous! I even have my own chaplain now—a really nice young fella."

We talked a bit about his family and the friends he was making in the nursing home.

"You're right, all these nurses do work together; sometimes the hospice nurses can manage the pain with special meds. It's a part of hospice. Have the nurses here call hospice if you have any problems with the medications or need something special. And I'll be visiting at least every two weeks, more if you'd like."

"I think my daughter might want to talk to you," he said. I said I'd phone her.

"She feels bad she can't have me at her house," he said. "But it's okay, I understand. She's working at a job she loves and she comes to see me regularly." Then he added quietly, "You know, I'm not afraid to die. I just don't know what I have to go through to get there."

Ah, now I know the very specific thing on his mind, I thought. *Something he'd been thinking about and was ready to talk about.* Most people are not that direct about the actual dying. I needed to know how specific he wanted me to be.

"That's a challenging thing to think about, isn't it? You make me think about what Woody Allen said about dying: 'I'm not afraid of dying. . . . I just don't want to be there when it happens.'[8] I love that!"

Mr. Edwards loved it too. He laughed and said, "Yep, I understand that. That's me, alright. Just don't know if it's gonna hurt, or what . . ."

"I'm glad you asked. Your nurses will give you more information about specific changes to expect and they will help you be comfortable physically. Some things that may happen are: your appetite may change, you may sleep more, and your feet and hands may feel cold to others but not to you. It's because the circulation slows down. Tell your nurse when you or your daughter are ready to look at the handout we have about what to expect. You are doing so well now, it may be a long time before those changes start. You may continue to be comfortable and not get weaker for a long time."

"What I've noticed being with people who are dying is that death is not the frightful thing people worry about. One woman expressed it this way: 'Death is usually a peaceful process . . . people just go to sleep.'"[9]

"And there's another thing: People have studied what happens when people are passing from this life to the next or when people have died and been revived. Many people report as they are dying that it's not even frightening; they feel calm and accepting of what is happening. Have you heard of any of those sorts of things?"

"I heard people see a bright light or a tunnel."

"Yes, some folk say they see a light of some kind, sometimes a tunnel or a border. Some people who have what they call 'near-death experiences' say similar things. It is interesting that a person's experience with a particular religion seems to shape what they see or experience; the experiences differ if they are Christian, Jewish, Muslim, or from a country where good and bad spirits are important to their belief. Often Christians believe they see Jesus, Catholics may say they see the Virgin Mary, and Jews sometimes call it a being of light or an angel. In some cultures, people expect to see the spirit of their loved ones."

"Another thing that may help is that, as I've been with dying people, if a person is not in physical pain (and you already know we can help with that) and if they are not having any emotional pain, the actual passing is peaceful. Many people find it a comfort when they have a faith that gives them comfort and answers about ultimate things."

"Ah, that's a good thing to know." Mr. Edwards said quietly. "Yep, my pain is not a problem now, and I have my friends and my family, so I guess I don't have anything to worry about there. What do you mean about 'emotional pain'?"

"Emotional pain is when you're frightened or worried; perhaps you've had a quarrel or there are bad feelings between you and someone else."

"Oh, no, I'm pretty easy to get along with; don't have any worries about things or people. And I've thought about it—don't have anybody I need to say 'sorry' to. I've been lucky that way; I'm pretty up front and make things right when they go wrong," he said with a smile. I could surely believe that.

"If you think of any of those things, emotional pains or worries, that you want to talk about, just call for me or the chaplain."

And then he really did not want to talk about that anymore. Instead, he began to tell me about his hobbies. He loved leather work, and he had the tools and equipment he needed so he could work on projects in his room. He was planning on making Christmas presents for his family.

A few days later, I met another new patient. Janice and I were alone on my first visit, having a relaxed conversation in her pleasant living room, talking about her family, her career, and her hobbies. I'd offered to talk with her about anything she wanted. Quietly she said, "I'm so afraid of what it's going to be like. You know, to actually die? How does it happen? Tell me everything about it." She obviously wanted a lot more information than Mr. Edwards had wanted; each individual has his or her own unique concerns.

"I certainly understand it can be a scary thought. I'm happy to talk to you about it. And I have some very good news for you. I've been with people when they were dying, and I've not seen it be a frightening process. Some say it's like getting weaker, very tired, and going to sleep. If there is any discomfort, the nurses will manage that and describe exactly what's happening."

"There are things we expect to happen. For instance, everything slows down; a person's circulation slows down, so hands and feet feel cold to those who touch you then. But you won't feel cold. You can plan ahead—you can write a plan, saying you want lights to be lowered, what music you'd like playing when you are relaxing near the end, who you want with you and those you *don't* want with you then! You are in charge! The nurses will tell you more and answer your questions too."

She relaxed a bit, it seemed. Likely she had been thinking about it for some time and wasn't sure what she'd learn—but she did want to know more about what to expect, and now she had the courage to ask. I thought to myself, *What a wonderful thing it is to be able to talk so openly about such a profound question.*

"Please say more . . ." Janice was eager to listen, so I cautiously shared some background on the studies and reported experiences.

"In the 1960s a young woman, a psychiatrist, came to the United States. She was sad and amazed to see how patients, families, and medical professionals did not want to talk about death. And she was shocked and concerned about how many folks spent their last days and died in hospitals without their family, and that children weren't allowed in the hospital to visit. She began to talk to medical people in training to help them be more aware of what was happening to people when they were seriously ill and how to better help them. You may even have heard of her: Dr. Elizabeth Kubler-Ross. She helped medical professionals become more willing to talk about grief, dying, and death with their patients." Janice seemed fascinated, wanting to know even more.

"Then Raymond Moody, a teacher and physician, talked to many people about the dying process. He thought it would help to learn what happened to folk who had been declared dead, perhaps because of an accident, and were revived. Many of them talked about having a 'near-death experience.' He compiled a list of fifteen things that are common for people to experience. Janice, have you heard about things people see when they are dying?"

Janice answered, "I've heard some of them see a light."

"Yes, now many people have studied near-death experiences, the closest thing studied to help us understand death. There are reports of a light or a being of light, an angel or a person they know; some believe it's Jesus. Sometimes there's a tunnel or a border of some kind. Most of the people Moody interviewed reported the experience as being calming, sometimes joyful, and usually peaceful."

"I've wanted to know, but I was afraid to ask anyone. Thank you, I'm not so scared; still, it's really strange. I still have a lot of questions."

"No one really knows for sure. I try to imagine what it must be like to have your life end. It's hard to understand and accept and sad to think of a person not being here anymore—his or her thoughts and memories gone. Still, the good news is that many people report it's not scary when you are comfortable physically as it actually happens."

"It's good to hear about that," Janice said quietly. "What do people say about the 'being' they see? Is it God?"

"People describe the bright light or being of light in different ways; some say it's Jesus, some say the Virgin Mary. Some say they see an angel or a spirit. Some people talk to the being or person they are seeing—a spouse, their father or mother, or other people. Sometimes they seem to be getting instruction from the people they see. Some people talk about events in their life—births, deaths, trips. And best of all, the patients often seem to be calmed by what they are seeing; they are not afraid. At that time it seems best to say 'How does that feel?,' 'Tell me more . . . ,' or to just be with the person, help them feel supported and loved."

"Some spiritual guides, researchers, and medical professionals believe those dying are actually seeing and interacting with others. Hospice nurse Maggie Callanan[10] calls these experiences 'nearing death awareness' and believes that 'they enter a state of expanded awareness.' Some social and medical scientists believe these things happen when a person's body is changing and becomes weaker when there is less oxygen, abnormal brain activity, or some other biological thing is happening. Some say it is a form of dementia; some folks believe people see what they expect or want to see."

"Thank you," Janice said. "I've had so many questions and didn't know if I wanted the answers. I think I can sleep better now. And I'll talk to my pastor about some of the other questions—about what happens after, where I'll go next, and what that's like."

"It's really important to think through what you believe with your pastor—or Marty, our chaplain—to think about what gives you strength and a safe feeling. We will be there to keep you as comfortable as possible. For now, remember the good things in your life, your work, the ways you have helped people, good relationships you've had, the things that give your life meaning. It's a time to thank folks, to ask for forgiveness or understanding, and to remember happiness and the things that give you peace. Each moment can be seen as more precious than it was before. Relax, meditate. Read if you like that, or listen to books on tape. Spend time with the people that matter. And ask us or the chaplain anything you wish."

Chapter Nine

Remembering

There are many beautiful and meaningful ways to remember and celebrate the lives of those we love. And there are almost no rights or wrongs when creating ways to remember loved ones. Each relationship is personal; some parts are private and some can be shared.

Families often ask their pastor, imam, priest, rabbi, or another spiritual leader to assist with services. Hospice chaplains and social workers are also available to help families as they create a wake, funeral, memorial, or graveside service. In addition to hospice, home funeral guides and death doulas or death midwives assist the family with final preparations and celebrations.[1]

My dad took me to the funerals of his colleagues when I was a child, modeling for me the appropriate behavior at a funeral. I saw bodies in caskets and urns with ashes. I observed the activities of the family, guests, pastor, and funeral directors—without dealing with grief for someone I knew. That was very wise of my dad; the experience was helpful to me then and as I worked with hospice patients and families.

Bereavement or grief begins when illness becomes chronic. It's sometimes called anticipatory grief. It intensifies when there is a terminal diagnosis. Many books and websites provide truly helpful information and guidance about grief in general, as well as specific kinds of grief.[2] More information is in the appendices.

In these stories you'll learn many ways to be involved in honoring those who have passed and supporting those who survive.

Remembering and Celebrating a Life

1. Create your own printed program for services using poems, songs, a brief life sketch, hobbies, artwork by the deceased, and important dates. Colored parchment paper is a nice touch; use full size, stapling or tying pages together or folded in half or quarters.

2. A "Life Celebration" can be created while the person lives; some folks write their own obituary and/or eulogy. I've created my own complete program!

3. Notify the local and hometown newspapers, alumni associations, and the folks in your book club, writers' group, garden club, honor societies, and homeowners' association.

4. Display scrapbooks, medals, honors, certificates, diplomas, and graduation caps.

5. Photos can be displayed in many ways—in a slideshow or video, framed, in albums, and arranged on a side table or on photo boards on easels.

6. Create a way for guests to write their own memories of the deceased using your word processor, possibly including some graphics. Plenty of room is available using half-pages with "Memories" in lovely script at the top and lines following for a personal message. Place them in a stack or a basket beside the guest book. The chaplain or a friend can read them as part of the service or they can be read by the guest from their place in the audience. Later they can be given to the family.

7. Give seed packets of flowers to folks as they leave the service; good choices include Forget-Me-Nots or the honored person's favorite flower.

8. Some churches have special times reserved during Christmas and New Years to remember sad events, called "Blue Christmas" or "Longest Night."[3]

9. Funeral homes offer personalized urns and pendants for ashes.

10. Social media provides opportunities for announcing a death and creating a memorial on the person's Facebook page and through blogs and websites. Stephanie Buck has written an overview of practical help and cautions about the management of a deceased person's Facebook page.[4] Candi Cann writes about new ways to memorialize the dead in very public ways using social media, tattoos, car decals, and funeral selfies in her book *Virtual Afterlives: Grieving the Dead in the Twenty-First Century*.[5]

11. Information is also available on social media to assist; some are businesses with fees involved (for example, Legacy Locker, BCelebrated).

12. Home funerals are increasingly popular. As in the past, some families consider caring for the body a precious gift to the deceased. With appropriate guidance, it is possible to have the loved one's body at home for several days after his or her death and to conduct a funeral there or at a gravesite. Green burials are available in some areas.[6] Even if death occurs in a hospital, convalescent facility, or hospice house, families have the right to choose to bring their loved one home. In addition to hospice care, home funeral guides, sometimes called death doulas or midwives, assist the family plan and carry out these services.[7]

13. On special days—Thanksgiving, Christmas, birthdays—make a toast to persons who have died. It's possible to use this opportunity to discuss your own plans and urge the family to think about their wishes and create advance directives for themselves. Michael Hebb began a movement to help folks create this type of opportunity to discuss end-of-life issues and advance directives; he calls it "Death over Dinner."[8]

14. Share stories with other families in special hospice events, often offered annually. End-of-life stories are available through other hospice sites and the National Hospice and Palliative Care Organization's website.

VIOLA JOHNSON, JEANETTE, PEGGY AND AL, THOMAS

There are wonderful ways to remember and celebrate a life.

Members of our hospice team often helped with memorial, funeral, and graveside services. And once a year we offered a community service, an evening of memories, poems, and thoughts from family members to honor our patients who had died in our care. This is a common practice in hospices.

Viola Johnson wrote poetry. I loved sitting on the sofa with her, listening to her read her own poems, which she artfully displayed in a leather scrapbook. When I heard she'd passed, I phoned her daughter: "Jan, I'm so sorry about your mom's death. She was a delightful woman. I have lovely memories of hearing her read her own poetry to me, sitting there on your sofa. Those poems will always mean a lot to you and your family. I think it would be lovely to display that scrapbook of her poems at the funeral home, next to the guest book, so folks can see it and read a poem or two. What do you think?"

"That's a wonderful idea. Thanks," Jan said. "I *will* bring the scrapbook, and I have an idea too—would you pick one of her poems to read as part of the service please? I'll tell the pastor and the funeral home people we want that included. And I'll bring some photo albums."

I agreed, of course, and a few days later, when I arrived at the funeral home, I identified myself to one of the funeral home directors: "Hello, I'm Karen from hospice; Mrs. Johnson's family has asked me to read a poem during the service. Who should I see?"

The director seemed really pleased: "Oh, good! Yes, go right up this hallway; you'll see the door to a small waiting room—the pastor is there. He'll be glad to see you." *That's nice*, I thought. *My goodness, he's so friendly.*

I found my way to the little room by the platform, and the pastor also greeted me very warmly. He did seem a bit harried, and asked me, "Do you know Mrs. Johnson?"

"Yes, I'm her social worker from hospice."

"Oh, good! I'm so glad you're here. Take as much time as you like."

He seemed overjoyed. *Interesting; these people are really friendly.* Then I discovered why. The relieved pastor told me: "The family called and asked me to conduct Mrs. Johnson's funeral. I said I'd be happy to. When I got here today I realized I've never seen this woman before! I don't know anything about her. There's a *different* Mrs. Johnson in my congregation; glad to know she's not deceased! Can you help me out and make them all feel better by talking about her? Read *two* poems and talk about her and her family please."

I read two poems from her scrapbook and reminisced about special things I know about her and about my visits with her; someone else who knew her gave the eulogy, and the pastor talked about spiritual things. I don't think most of the folks listening even had a clue about the mix up.

Jeanette was a volunteer with "Reach to Recovery," the American Cancer Society's program for breast cancer patients and survivors. A survivor herself and a positive, energetic woman, she offered survivors a special celebration at the end of their funeral or memorial. She invited other survivors to join her, standing in a circle on the grass outside the funeral home or in the cemetery, often inviting family members and the hospice team to join them. They held helium-filled pink balloons on pink strings while they shared memories of their friend. Then the balloons were released and we watched them float away, each person remembering their friend, privately thinking of their own beliefs about death and the hereafter. Beautiful memories can help us manage the grief we feel in loss and create a good new memory.

Peggy and Al were a dynamic duo obviously in love; they enjoyed telling our team about their mid-life romance. Because of a blood transfusion Peggy received during back surgery, both eventually became infected with the HIV virus, which then developed into full-blown AIDS in both of them. Al was our patient for a few weeks; it was hard for everyone to manage his illness while realizing how ill Peggy was also and knowing she would likely die soon. Peggy was devastated when Al died; she adored him and blamed herself for his death.

Peggy and her kids planned several unique things for Al's service in their church, and she was hurt and angry when the pastor said he didn't believe "The Dance" by Garth Brooks[9] was appropriate for a church funeral and wouldn't let her include it. Peggy told me, "My family knows they are to have my service in a place that will let them play that song. It was our song; it really told our story."

I promised her I'd help and nothing would stop us from using that song. When she passed, I created her personal memorial service program, eight pages on 9" × 12" pale gold parchment-like paper. The family choose several poems, we listed the name of each family member, told a bit of her love story, and included the words to "The Dance."

Everything was well-prepared and going smoothly. I decided to take a back road from our office to the small town where the memorial was to be held; even with the hills, valleys, and curves I'd calculated my time to get there before folks began arriving. The morning of Peggy's service, I was going faster than my usual cautious three miles over the posted speed when I saw a sheriff's car traveling toward me, past me, and then saw it in my rearview mirror as he whipped around, turned on his light, drove up behind me, and indicated I was to stop. I stopped and pulled out my driver's license and retrieved my registration.

"Do you know how fast you were going?" he asked

"Too fast, I know. Usually I travel just about the speed limit—honest. I'm really in a hurry—on my way to a funeral." *Yeah, right*, he was likely thinking. "See this stack of papers on the passenger seat?" I continued, indicating the seventy-five packets of gold parchment-like paper. "Those are the programs for the funeral—honest. It's a hospice memorial actually; I'm their hospice social worker—and *I'm* conducting the memorial service. They're waiting for these programs," I hurried on. "They need to be there *now* while people are arriving. The service is at 11:00. Twenty minutes . . ."

He didn't seem impressed; I decided he needed more information. "It's for Peggy Cane. You probably know Peggy; she and Al, except he died a little while ago, they owned the appliance shop on the highway." *Ah! Recognition, he'd known them. Thank goodness.* Likely he also saw the tears of frustration in my eyes.

"Officer," I began again, deciding to try one more tug on his heartstrings, "please, I need to get there with the programs, my team and the funeral directors are waiting for me." Then I had an inspiration: "I know, you could follow me there, let me give them the programs—and *then* give me a ticket."

"Oh, just go. Watch your speed, okay?"

The service was really difficult for everyone; it helped that we used many personal references to Al and Peggy and their special relationship and their too-short time together. Their children doubly grieved. It is still a joy for me to remember them. The eight-page program included quotes from family and friends and, of course, the words to "The Dance," which was played at the service this time.

Thomas was a rather quiet man. The only time I saw him really animated was when he talked about his volunteering at the fire department in his small town. When he passed, he was "carried" (a great Southern term) from the church where the funeral service was held to the cemetery by the local fire truck, with his fellow volunteer firemen friends standing on every available space on the truck. Town folk lined the streets and then walked behind the truck to the tiny cemetery.

There are many unique and beautiful ways to remember a life.

LITTLE JIMMY

"I want to be with my daddy."

Our hospice assisted a young family when Jim, a husband, father, and son, was terminally ill. A few days after his funeral, Janet, the young mother, called us about her five-year-old son: "Please come talk to my Jimmy; he wants to die and be with his father."

Jim and the family had been stunned when he was diagnosed with late-stage cancer. Jim bravely battled his cancer. He was on our hospice program for a very short time. The team worked intensely to help with many visits by the nurse, the aide, the chaplain, and myself. He died at age forty-two. We comforted the family and helped them create a memorial service with a hand-fashioned brochure of poems, hymns, and his short life story; our chaplain conducted the service.

I met with Jim's widow the afternoon that she called us about Jimmy. She was frightened and didn't know what to do for him. We met in a quiet park in her small town; she didn't want to talk where Jimmy could hear. His grandma was caring for him at home.

"When Jim died," Janet said, "we told Jimmy that his daddy was an angel now, and that he was with God in heaven. We told him that he misses us, but he's happy, and one day we'll be with him again. We even hung a Christmas angel from the ceiling as a reminder that his daddy was an angel and with the angels in heaven. We said, 'Daddy is okay now, he isn't sick anymore.'"

I reassured her, "You were trying hard to help Jimmy understand what you believe about his father now; you wanted him to feel better. You had reasons for each thing you said. Did something specific happen?" I asked her.

"What happened was he decided he wanted to be with his dad!" she said. "This morning I found him standing on his dad's bed, dressed in Jim's shirt and hat—can you imagine what that looked like? First, it seemed funny, then we saw he had his dad's gun on the bed beside him. Jim's mom was with me, and we panicked. We grabbed him and said, 'What are you doing?'"

"He got really upset," Janet was agitated with herself now, recounting the story. "He was screaming and crying, 'Let me go. Let me go . . .'"

"Sweetie, what's wrong? You can't touch the gun . . ."

"I want to be with my daddy, I want to be an angel too."

"Yes," I said, "and Jimmy doesn't know what death is, so the best thing he could think of was to be with his dad whatever it took. He thought that if he died too, he'd be with Jim. It's very hard to deal with your own grief and his too."

She sobbed and I held her. Then I said, "That must have been so frightening for you."

"I just don't know how to manage all this. I'm so sad myself, and I have to be a mom first. I know that he doesn't understand any of this, I know that too. What can I do?"

"It does feel so sad—for everybody: for you, Jim's mom, and for Jimmy."

Calmly I talked to her and I was thinking how frightening this all was. Fear is often at the basis of many other emotions—anger, discouragement, depression. Janet did not know how she would manage, emotionally, as a mom—or financially either.

"Janet, this is such a big load for you to carry. It's hard enough for us adults to manage through all this grief. There's no way for him to understand. He doesn't really know what death is, can't think it all through. I'm guessing he didn't even realize if he went to heaven with his dad, he wouldn't have you."

"I've read one woman's description of what this kind of thing is like for kids. She says it's kind of like being hit by a lightning bolt—out of the blue, devastating, like a world torn apart. She says it creates 'panic, pain, terror, and confusion.' Her name is Maxine Harris and she's written a book titled *The Loss that Is Forever*.[10] Perhaps we can find that book for you. We know Jimmy really didn't understand how sick his daddy was; there would be no way for him to understand. Even when you try to explain something like that, he doesn't understand the words."

Janet bowed her head. She took long slow breaths. "You know, I did say something like, 'Jimmy, sweetie, if you went to daddy, then I'd be alone. Grandma and I need you here with us.' He let me hold him; he calmed down and said he wanted to wear daddy's shirt for a while. We rolled up the sleeves, tied a belt around his middle, and he played a bit, then laid down and slept for a while. That's when I called you."

"You see, Janet," I said, "you did a wonderful thing. You thought of a way to help him stay connected to his dad with the shirt, and you took time to cuddle him and help him feel close to you. Good job." And I continued: "The chaplain and I are happy to meet with you and with Jimmy—together and separately. And I've been thinking about how we can help him—and you— long term. There's a really good family counseling center nearby, and they have a counselor for children. She would work mostly with Jimmy, but she'd help you too. And there's a support group called "Life After Loss" sponsored by the American Cancer Society—Jim's hospice nurse Cindy is one of the facilitators. There's no charge for the ACS group and it meets in the early evening so you could go after work. The counseling center charges based on your income. How do those things sound to you?"

Janet reacted right away: "Oh, wonderful. It all sounds good. I'm glad the chaplain and you are still here for us. We loved the way you printed the funeral program just for Jim, I'll keep it forever; it has his favorite Bible verses and poems. Still, I know I'm going to need someone to talk to many times—I'd love to be part of something with other wives. Could Jim's mother come with me too?"

"Absolutely. You can go together or separately. We'll check to see if they have child care while you're there. I've written down the phone number and address of the counseling center. What else can I do to help? Are you comfortable calling them or do you want me to call and get you started?"

"I can do it," she said. Still, tears came. She was so exhausted, dealing with her own grief and so concerned about Jimmy. "I don't know what to say to him when he wakes up."

"You can help him. Lots of hugs and listening. Tell him you're really sad too, and you won't go away, and that you don't want him to go away. Tell him you'd be sad like he is now, missing his dad, if he went away. Sit down with him today and ask him to talk to you about his dad. Remember, kids think concretely in black and white. You can write some of the words he uses about Jim on 4" × 6" cards. Write in big letters, using colored pens. Today or another day, put those 4" × 6" cards each on a page of a scrapbook and have Jimmy draw pictures about those words. For example, for the word 'love' he may draw a heart. Use 'mom,' 'dad,' and 'school.' What else do you think you could include?"

"Ahh, snapshots—especially ones of Jimmy with Jim, and the program from the funeral. I can think of lots of things. That will help him—I think it will help me. Maybe I'll make one for myself . . ."

"Good job. Good thinking!"

"I have one more idea," I said. "Let him wear Jim's shirt a bit, maybe just in the house to keep it special. Of course, you'll need to have him take it off so you can wash it. Get him used to not wearing it, then tell him you'll put it on a 'big man hanger' and hang it in his closet. Tell him he can wear it when he grows up. Do you think that might help?"

"That's a good idea. I'll feel it out as I go. Thanks."

"Janet, I'm going to see the librarian here and ask her to purchase two DVDs for kids—one is about serious illness, one about death, grief, and loss. Then they'll be available to you and the community. They are written by a hospice nurse, Christy Whitney.[11] And there is help from *Sesame Street* for kids who are grieving.[12] There may be other books there to help also. Try these things and call when I can help."

"Check the website for the Dougy Center," I also suggested. "They focus on grief in children. Here's a description they use that I like:

> The most basic feeling of loss for a child is that of fear. Fear and uncertainty about: What happened? Who will die next? Will my other parent die? Who will take care of me? Where will I go if I die? Why did it happen? And, most especially, Will I die?[13]

I'll have Jim's hospice nurse Cindy call you about the ACS support group. You will be alright. Call us anytime."

I think of her even now, dealing with her own terrible griefs—first, the diagnosis, then months of caring for Jim, trying to involve the little one, and trying to understand what he was thinking and feeling. Sometimes the grief and the caregiving can seem overwhelming; still, helping Jimmy helped her too. It required her looking outside herself—and she had our help to find ways to work through this terrible loss and its challenges to her family.

Surviving and Thriving after Loss

1. Our first duty is to take care of ourselves, then we have the strength and the will to reach out again to others.
2. Be gentle with yourself. Let yourself feel the feelings; name them and acknowledge that they are reasonable, whatever they are. They reflect your memories of the person you loved and your dreams, hopes, fears, and disappointments.
3. Remember the love. Celebrate the life.
4. Do something active.
5. Talk about it. Feel. Cry. Laugh. Mourn.
6. Write about it in a diary or journal, daily or when you feel like it.
7. Ask for help. Look for help in your community and on the Internet (for example, AARP, American Cancer Society, Alzheimer's Association, Parkinson's Foundation, ALS Association).
8. Seek help from friends, professionals, and support groups.

9. Make plans for today, tomorrow, next month, and next year.
10. At holidays, do something you did with the person you lost and do something new to create new traditions.
11. Read. Read books about grief; read books to distract yourself.
12. Listen to others who have lost.
13. Enjoy your new self.

Chapter Ten

Mixed Feelings about End-of-Life Care

Physicians, counselors, nurses, social workers, therapists, chaplains, and others in the helping professions choose careers in which they can help people be healthy physically, emotionally, mentally, and spiritually. When illness occurs, their goal is to help patients get better—and be comfortable. Ideally, they listen carefully to their patients, use their best training and skills to choose and administer the best course of action, provide complete information about how various treatment options can help, and describe possible negative side effects. Their focus is quality of life, and they diagnose, treat, and manage symptoms so that patients *feel* better while working to *get* better.

When severe symptoms (for example, pain, nausea, trouble breathing, anxiety, depression, not eating) diminish a person's quality of life, a palliative care team can be consulted to focus on managing symptoms, even when there is no terminal diagnosis. Palliative care can begin at any time symptoms are difficult.

Hospice care can continue that palliative (comfort) care when a patient becomes terminally ill, when no treatment for cure is available or desired. At that point, patients usually are seeking quality of life rather than a quantity of time. Six full months of care are available in hospice—and, sad to say, 40.5 percent of patients who used hospice in 2016 waited to choose hospice until the last two weeks, and a close to one-third (27.9 percent) waited until the last week of life. [1]

Some people tell me they think hospice is a really good thing—for later. *Much later.* Why do so many patients, caregivers, families, and some health care professionals wait? Some of the reasons are:

- Life is precious and people don't want to talk about death, choosing to concentrate on getting better, continuing treatment, and hoping and planning for a cure.
- They don't understand hospice or its benefits.
- They believe it's only for the last few days of life instead of a full six months.
- Some believe it's only for cancer patients, but "nearly two-thirds of patients were admitted . . . with non-cancer primary diagnoses."[2]
- They don't want to go to a place called "hospice." Hospice is not a place, it's a kind of care provided by a multidisciplinary team brought to them where they live. Some hospices do have a separate hospice house or a dedicated unit in a medical facility, used if care becomes too difficult at home.
- They believe they can't afford it, not understanding that hospice is a benefit of Medicare, Medicaid, VA Benefits, and many other insurance plans. It's the least expensive way for patients, families, and the government to provide care at the end of life, usually avoiding multiple visits to their doctor's office, ER visits, and hospital stays.
- Patients fear a loss of independence. When cared for by hospice, they learn the blessings of interdependence between the patient, the caregivers, and the hospice team.
- They don't want to "give up," not realizing that hospice is not about giving up but about choosing expert end-of-life care focusing on quality of life. Some patients improve and sign off hospice services; they can request them when needed at a later time.
- They believe they have to have a DNR (do not resuscitate). Patients remain in control of their own decisions. They can create a physician orders for sustaining life form (POLST)[3] with their physician outlining exactly what they want and what they don't want. Often patients choose to have a DNR but can change their minds.
- Their physicians do not describe the benefits or do not refer patients to hospice.
- Some physicians are not comfortable discussing hospice with patients.
- Some patients will continue to fight to live without hospice care, no matter how well the benefits are presented to them.
- Some patients and families avoid news they don't want to hear.

Sometimes aggressive treatment diminishes the quality of life as a cost of living longer. Dr. Atul Gawande, a surgeon and advocate for making good end-of-life decisions, writes about watching the physical decline of some patients and his own father. Both of his parents were also physicians, and he and they often talked about patient care. In his recent book, *Being Mortal:*

Medicine and What Matters in the End,[4] he describes a default setting for physicians as focusing on the next best treatment.

"I learned about a lot of things in medical school," Dr. Gawande writes, "but mortality wasn't one of them."[5] He says it was difficult to accept that his father might not recover; later recognizing that "death is not a failure. Death is normal."[6] Dr. Gawande and his parents realized that his father's treatments were becoming debilitating and that his quality of life was decreasing with no hope of recovery. He learned more about hospice care when he visited patients in their homes with a hospice nurse; later, he and his parents chose home hospice care for his father. Gawande describes how, with hospice care, his father stabilized, his symptoms were better managed, his decline slowed, and he had many good days again, able to do some of his favorite things: watching football and eating ice cream, commenting, "We witnessed for ourselves the consequences of living for the best possible day today instead of sacrificing time now for time later."[7]

Pain management and conversations about end-of-life choices can be difficult for some physicians and other health care professionals, especially those who were in school before they were required to study those topics. Continuing education courses available to them include pain management, symptom management, end-stages of diseases, and end-of-life issues. And there are programs available to assist physicians be more comfortable talking about end-of-life decisions, such as Clear Conversations (Kaiser) and the Doc2Doc Program from Compassion and Choices.[8]

There are even mnemonic (memory) tools to assist with cultural awareness about advance care planning offered by the American Academy of Hospice and Palliative Medicine (AAHPM) and Hospice and Palliative Nurses Association (HPNA). They use the phrase A REFLECTION: Allow, Reflect, Empathize, Facilitate, Listen, Engage, Compassionately Bridge, Trust, Inquire, Open, and Name Needs.[9]

"'Quality of life for seriously ill patients over extending life as long as possible' was favored by 96 percent of a sample of 500 physicians."[10] Still, 42 percent of them had some hesitations about comfort care, responding that they were concerned about focusing on palliative/comfort care and not continuing to work on curing the patient. Retired family practice physician Ken Murray provides some interesting insights about the end-of-life decisions made by doctors for themselves: "What's unusual about them is not how much treatment they get compared to most Americans, but how little . . . they go gently . . . they know enough about modern medicine to know its limits."[11]

Each of us has options for end-of-life care, and medical professionals have a personal and professional duty to provide the best information available, including the pluses and minuses of treatment, and then support the patients' rights to decide for themselves about their care. The physician, patient, and family need to discuss advance directives and honor the patient's wishes. Sophia's story in chapter 11 provides questions and answers about how families can work with each other and with medical professionals to understand options and make good choices.

Most physicians and other health care professionals are sensitive to patient needs, fears, and questions. Some have a hard time talking with patients and family members when there is no more hope of a cure. Dr. Jamison's story shows how he became more comfortable with difficult conversations.

DR. JAMISON

"I just can't say the word 'hospice' to my patients."

In my role as hospital discharge planner before I chose to work in hospice, I visited, encouraged, and assessed every patient considered "high risk," including those with Medicare or Medicaid coverage, and all patients who had a life-limiting illness. Sandra Thompson, in her seventies with late-stage cancer, had been receiving treatment from Dr. Jamison for some time.

"I just don't feel good most of the time," she told me. "I'm so weak, and it's getting harder to do everyday things. Then there's Charlie—he's not good either."

"It's hard to not have energy. That can be very discouraging," I said. "There are several community programs that may help when you get home— Meals on Wheels, emergency devices, support groups, and homemaker services. Some are free, some have a fee, and sometimes the cost is based on your income."

I described the services, and she said, "Yes, I think I want that emergency device I can wear. I'll feel safer. Maybe we should order one for Charlie too. He likes to go for walks, and I'd not be so worried if he had a way to get help if he fell or got lost. And I'll try the meals program; we'll see how that works out. I'll talk to my daughter about some of the other things."

"Your daughter can call me if she likes," I said, giving her my card. "I'll leave the information about Meals on Wheels, the emergency device, and the other programs. You or your daughter can call them. I'll phone you when you get home and we'll talk again."

We talked a few more minutes, and then I wished her well and said goodbye. Next, I went to the nurses' station and entered my assessment in Mrs. Thompson's chart, including a question for her physician: "Dr. Jamison, do you think this patient may be appropriate for hospice?"

I knew this kind, gentle, young physician. He had many senior citizens in his practice, and message was to encourage him to consider making a hospice referral when he thought the time was right. I wrote notes like that on patient charts because you don't *tell* the doctor what to do, you *suggest.* In the past, there had been no response from Dr. Jamison about my hospice referrals.

The next day I saw him at the nurses' station and asked if we could talk for a few minutes; he knew why I wanted to talk. We stepped to a quiet place in the hallway, and he said, "I know . . . I know. I *know* hospice is a good thing. I don't have more treatments or any possibility of a cure to offer her, but I just can't say *that word* to my patients or their families."

"Ah, I can certainly understand that," I said. "It's not easy to talk about 'comfort care' when you and they want so much more. They're waiting to hear you say you can fix things. It's hard to know when to focus only on comfort and symptom management."

"Yes, it is, and I do know this patient is ready for comfort care. She won't live long. I just think if I talk to her or her family about hospice they'll feel like I'm giving up on her."

Ah, there it is, I thought. *He believes hospice can give her good care and can help the family cope, he's just not comfortable talking about it or even saying the word. It seems too difficult—easier to have her keep coming to his office where he can continue to listen to her, talk to her and her husband, and prescribe medications to relieve her symptoms. There, he can try to help them feel more secure. Nobody wants to face what is really happening.*

"Perhaps," I said, "it would help if you told them what you can *give* them at this point, describing the care without saying the word hospice until later. You could say something like:

> **Here's what I want to give you:** a nurse coming to your home on a regular basis and on call for emergencies and whatever medical equipment and medications to help you be comfortable and keep your symptoms under control. You'll have a social worker, like Karen, who can connect you to community resources and sit and listen when that helps. The hospice chaplain can visit in your home, and a nurse's aide can visit a couple of hours a day when you need help with personal care. Best thing is, it won't cost anything to you or your family. It's part of your Medicare benefits.

> **This is the best care I can give you right now.** The folks are licensed health care professionals; they know how to take good care of you and make sure you're comfortable. They specialize in treating symptoms, especially pain. They'll help your caregivers—Mr. Thompson and your daughter. I'd like to have Karen come to your room and talk to you about this kind of care. It's called hospice. You can have your daughter come for that visit too if you like. I'll write an order for a hospice referral in your chart.

He was listening intently, and I continued: "You'll find your own way to describe all the who, what, when, where, why, and how things about hospice. It's easier on the patient and their family than frequent ER visits, ICU admissions, or hospital or nursing home stays.[12] The care she needs can be given at home, and Medicare pays for it. You can continue to be her doctor if you wish, consulting with the hospice physician. Studies show that some patients actually live longer and have a better quality of life once they are admitted to hospice than similar patients who don't have hospice care."[13]

I could see the relief on his face. He wanted what was best for this patient and her family. He was beginning to see that he could feel good about giving them hospice. Soon, using his own description, he talked with her and her daughter, then placed the referral to hospice on her chart. He began referring other patients to hospice too. He had just not known how to present the idea in a positive way. Having something to *give* them now was a blessing to him also.

Chapter Eleven

Making Good End-of-Life Decisions

Choosing the right end-of-life option is more likely when you have good information about the choices available and create advance directives so your wishes will be known and honored. The goal is good continuity of care.

- Palliative care, now a medical specialty, is a good choice for management of distressing symptoms (for example, pain, nausea, anorexia, breathing difficulties, anxiety, depression) even when there is no terminal diagnosis.
- Palliative care, also sometimes called comfort care, is the focus of both "palliative care" and "hospice care."
- Hospice care is for terminally ill patients when no more treatment is available or they want to stop treatment. It is most helpful when chosen early enough to have the full six months of care available.

It wasn't so long ago, up to the mid-1800s,[1] that almost everyone was cared for and died at home. As medical technology advanced, people began to rely on aggressive care—CPR, the emergency room, an intensive care unit, hospital stays, and rehabilitation. Individuals who say they don't want to rely on tubes, machines, and heroic measures past the time when they have what they consider acceptable quality of life often die in hospitals with major equipment keeping them alive.[2] Understanding options for care and completing advance directives can help folks have the care they want and not endure the treatments they don't want at the end of life. Advance directives include choosing an agent, sometimes called a representative or surrogate, to carry out their wishes when they can't speak for themselves. The Washington State Medical Association's brochure[3] asks: "Who will decide if you can't?"

Advance directives can be found on websites in each state. There is another vital form: actual doctor's orders. These are called physician orders

for life-sustaining treatment (POLST or MOLST). These are useful for everyone and vital for frail or terminally ill persons. The doctor keeps a copy and
one goes with the patient. It's a good idea to have a copy available on your
person when you travel, posted in your home, and in the hands of your
personal medical agent.

SOPHIA AND HER DAD

"How do I talk to my dad about his illness?"

"I just can't say the words."

"Which words?" I asked.

"I can't tell him he's not going to get better. It seems to me he's getting
worse, but I don't know. How do I talk to my dad about his illness?"

"Ah, that is hard. What does he tell you about how he feels?"

"He says that he's tired and he knows things aren't good. But now he tells
me his doctor says he's got another treatment that might help."

"How do you feel about that?"

"Of course, we all want to do anything and everything that will really
help."

"Hmm, then you and he need to find out if that treatment will really help.
My first suggestion is that you and he ask his doctor what the major problems
are and what options are available. If you'd like we can meet at your break,
have something hot to drink, and talk more about your concerns. I'll meet
you at the hospital coffee shop; you tell me the time."

Sophia was a volunteer at our hospital, and I'd gotten into this conversation while my husband was filling out forms for outpatient surgery. I told her
I was thinking of volunteering there too, one thing led to another, and she
learned I'd been a hospice social worker. I often meet people who have a
curiosity about hospice but don't really know much about it. It's my goal to
demystify hospice, and Sophia was a good candidate to hear more.

Later, sipping steaming cups of tea, Sophie said, "I guess I'm really
having trouble accepting that he's so sick; I'm not ready to let him go. I do
want the doctor to be able to help him if he can. We've tried so many
things—surgery, chemo, radiation, pills. He's so tired out and he doesn't feel
good a lot of the time. He's not himself . . ."

Then she was weeping quietly. I waited and then she said, "It's always
been hard to talk to him about serious things."

"Tell me about your Dad—when he was well . . ."

She smiled and said, "He was a quiet and strong man, he loved his work,
helped to create a good home for his family. He loved the out-of-doors, loved
playing games inside and out. There were times when he quietly sat in his

study reading or working on his stamp collection, and there were active family times with my brothers and I, when we were little, and older too."

"He was so strong and secure. He's always been active and still gentle with my mom and us kids. He listened and helped us with whatever was happening in our lives, but he didn't like to talk about himself—about how he was feeling." She was quiet for a moment, then said, "He's been lonely since mom died. We stay involved with him; we're all grieving mom. He was so good with her when she was sick, so we have those lovely memories of that too. He was right on top of things, talking to her doctor, getting the equipment she needed, giving her meds . . ."

"Sophia, I'm going to suggest ways you can help him *stay* in charge of his life. I think it will be good for you and your dad and any other siblings to have a serious talk. Start with a family dinner maybe. You can begin by thanking him for caring for your mom and talking to her doctor. Let him know you're concerned about his health, that you'd all like to get more information, and talk to his doctor. After you've talked together, you can arrange for a family conference with the doctor."

"It sounds like a good thing, except we can't bother the doctor like that."

"Sophia, your dad's doctor is really his employee. The doctor's job is to do what's best for your dad. He needs your dad's okay for any new treatment, for any decisions, and hopefully he wants the family's cooperation and support. Medicare now pays the doctor for consults like that."

"Please give me your email address and I'll send you information about websites that will be a big help." I took a small tablet from my purse, wrote down her email address, and began jotting down ideas for Sophia.

"I'll give a list of questions to ask the doctor, we'll talk a bit about the choices you have, and you can go to the websites for more information. Right now this may seem overwhelming, but the information on these websites is wonderfully helpful. Take a little time to print the documents and the guidelines, give yourself time to read and absorb the information, and put it all in a folder. You may want to make copies for your brothers. You will feel more confident in moving ahead. Using this information, my husband and I have brought our advance directives up to date, the attorney made changes in our original documents—and I now carry a copy with us when we travel, and we have them on file at our primary care physician's office and our hospital. We also take them with us when we travel to see our daughter and her husband in Australia. You never know . . ."

"Yes, I realize our whole family needs to make sure things are in order . . ." she said.

"Sophia, there are a lot of people urging individuals and families to talk candidly about illness, choices, and decisions. There are many books written about it, and websites, lots of good information. One doctor calls it 'Having the Conversation.'"

Angelo Volandes, MD,[4] journalist Ellen Goodwin,[5] and many other advocates for quality of life are encouraging families to talk about what they want to happen when they face a traumatic injury or serious illness. Information and guidelines about beginning to talk about this are available on the internet through "The Conversation Project."[6]

"When you get home, go on the internet and take some time to get acquainted with the information we've talked about; that will help you use the questions I'll give you—and you can add more. You can help your dad talk about what's happening to him and help him clarify how he feels and what he wants. He may actually be relieved to honestly look at his illness and his choices. A professor friend of mine calls this kind of thing Q & C—questions and concerns.[7] You can share the list with your brothers and they can add their own version of Q & C. Then talk to your dad. Use my list or create your own Q & C list for the doctor, then ask for a family conference and get some answers. Some doctor's offices also have a social worker or a 'navigator' who will help you and connect you with resources. This list will help you get started . . ."

"Okay, I'll check out the information on the websites and talk to the boys . . ."

That conversation was a lot to take in, but Sophia was listening, wanting more information. I continued: "If and when your dad decides he doesn't' want any more treatment for a cure, or the doctor says there is not more treatment he recommends, you can ask that he refer your dad to hospice. Talk to him about it, and you can ask the doctor for hospice yourself when you think the time is right and the doctor doesn't suggest it."

"A hospice nurse will go to your dad's home and do an assessment—you'll want to be there. If they believe your dad is appropriate for hospice care, they will contact his doctor. When the doctor agrees, he'll sign papers to make the hospice care official. It's a Medicare entitlement; there usually is no cost to you or your dad."

"With some hospices, your dad's physician can still be his primary care doctor, conferring with the hospice doctor as an end-of-life specialist. Your dad would have the care in his home—nurse visits, a nurse aide when he needs that, a social worker, a chaplain, and all the medication and medical equipment he needs."

Sophia said, "I'm so relieved. I just didn't know where to begin. . . . Thank you."

Here is some of the information I shared with Sophia:

- *The Conversation Project*: basic information, guidebooks, examples.[8]
- *Let's have dinner and talk about death (Death over Dinner)*.[9]
- *Caring Community/Caring Conversations*: provides a guide for family members to talk about end-of-life topics and decisions.[10]

- *End of Life, Washington*:[11] easy-to-understand and download basic information about advance directives that you can complete and have notarized or take to your attorney; usually you can find a similar site in any state.

Questions to Ask Your Doctor about Your Illness and Your Choices

1. Please tell me my exact diagnosis.
2. How do people usually die when they have what I have?
3. How long do people usually live with this illness?
4. What treatments are there that may help, and what are their negative side effects?
5. Am I at risk for stroke, heart attack, or other problems?
6. If I was your mother or father, what would you do next?
7. How will I know when to ask for hospice care and will you help me get it?
8. What are the signs of dying from this disease?
9. If you have any printed material about that, please share it with me.
10. When the time comes, can you support me in staying at home as long as possible?

Important: If your doctor is unwilling to talk to you and answer these questions or is unwilling to support you in your choices, you need to find a doctor who will. Take good notes.

How to Be an Effective Advocate for Yourself or a Family Member

1. Practice good preventative care, see your physician(s) regularly, and follow their advice. Urge family members to do the same.
2. Learn about options for medical care in critical and end-of-life situations and create advance directives; have them notarized; distribute them to your physicians, hospital, and family members; keep a file in a safety deposit box; and carry copies when you travel.
3. When you have an illness or accident, seek treatment and follow the treatment plan.
4. Keep a journal, by date, about illnesses, accidents, symptoms, and severity (e.g., 0–10 scale), physician appointments with questions for the physician and their directions, record medications taken, record results.
5. Keep your family informed and involved.

6. When your health worsens, see the physician; possibly ask for a family conference.
7. Comfort care is a part of medical care. You may request a palliative care consult with a specialist when symptoms don't improve or worsen.
8. When illness or symptoms worsen, talk to your physician about end-of-life care choices.
9. When an illness become life-limiting/terminal, request a hospice care consult.
10. Make your own choices about your care in conference with your family and physicians.

Chapter Twelve

Reflections

MEDICAL SOCIAL WORK

The most amazing, exhausting, and fulfilling job.

Yes, most of my patients died, and yes, I chose to become a hospice social worker after many other interesting social work positions: I'd worked at a residential treatment center for kids (not an easy task), and I'd worked in adoptions and loved it, partly because my kids are adopted. I was a discharge planner in county hospitals and private hospitals, very enjoyable, meeting patients and families, encouraging and supporting them, then connecting them to helpful community resources, including hospice. Then I chose to work in hospice care.

My father and I cared for my mom through her ten-year cancer experience and death. She was diagnosed with breast cancer in 1974. She had treatment, kept active, even took an eight-week trip to Europe. During those ten years she had cancer we lived in Washington State and she lived in Michigan, and we visited back and forth as much as we could. When we lived in the Republic of the Philippines for three years, she and my dad spent two months with us there—she was on crutches, which did not stop her. She spent two months in our home when we returned from the Philippines near the end of her journey: she was able to attend my college graduation. She then went home and died three weeks later.

Hospice was just coming into its own as an encouraging and positive idea in the field of medicine and social work. The first hospice opened in 1974; Congress first approved funding for hospice in 1984. My mother died in 1983; we were not offered hospice care.

Fortunately, I'd learned some skills in understanding and working with grief, loss, and dying during the "death and dying" movement led by its guru Elizabeth Kubler-Ross.[1] I'd read her books, attending lectures she gave in Fort Worth, and was intrigued by her focus on having the family more involved in the care of dying patients, especially in medical facilities. My major was social services, I earned a social work license, then attended graduate school, studying sociology. I knew someday I wanted to be part of the world of hospice. What I learned about grief has helped in all areas of my social work experience, including later as director of patient services for a regional office of the American Cancer Society.

People have asked me, "Why would you do this work?" My answer: It truly is a blessing to be a useful part of people's lives, to listen to their stories, help them talk about the meaningful things they've done, encourage them to connect or reconnect with family and friends, say their thank yous, and make amends when necessary before they say their final goodbyes. I enjoyed being someone who heard their questions and concerns about being so ill, helped relieve their anxieties and suffering, guided them in ways to cope, and assisted with very practical needs.

People asked me why, but mostly they wanted to know *how* I could do it. I dove in head first, happy to be on that particular front line. Then I slowed down and handled it like this:

- *Taking it one day at a time.* My work was officially limited to forty hours per week. Some calls involved nights and weekends, and one week a month I was on 24/7 call. I did what needed doing mostly during regular hours and compensated other times.
- *Pacing myself,* taking time off after an especially difficult visit, stopping at a café for a coffee and some downtime.
- *Preparing and decompressing.* On my thirty- to forty-five-minute ride to work each morning, I prepared emotionally, thinking of the folks I'd be visiting that day, and I tried to chill, usually with Neil Diamond, on the drive home.
- *Being creative with vacations.* I had three weeks' vacation annually, and I'd take them one week at a time, adding paid days off to have the Friday before and the Monday after my vacation weeks off.
- *Continuing other interests.* During one vacation each year I went to conferences relating to my sociological interests (for example, cross-cultural issues, diversity training, academic study of religion and belief systems). That new information provided more insights into my hospice work. I spent one vacation a year with my wild and wacky friend, Nan.
- *Balancing the emotional weight of hospice work,* teaching evening courses in sociology, and attending or conducting workshops.

- *Sharing ideas, questions, challenges, and frustrations* with other team members.
- *Reading a lot* about death and dying, hospice, family dynamics, and belief systems.
- *Reading about other things.*
- *Escaping into films, drama, daydreaming* . . . other ways to learn about life.
- *Writing* about all kinds of things.

The work wasn't easy. However, it was the most amazing, exhausting, and fulfilling job I have ever had—not counting childrearing. Writing about the experiences has been cathartic for me; I have *needed* to think and write about what I did. All the resources I had were called into play and I made those moments the best they could be.

No, I'm not co-dependent. I really bristled when that was suggested—and it was. It is important to find balance. But please, there is nothing wrong and everything right with enjoying helping people. The term co-dependency alludes to helping others to the point of hurting yourself. I didn't do that. I emotionally put things on what I called "the shelf" so I could get on with the next patient, the next family. Occasionally the shelves got full and I was sad and weighted down. But not often, and it was worth it.

Most of the time I loved the work. In those moments working with the patient, the caregivers, and my colleagues, we were all living *in* the moment, attuned to each other and making a difference. Sometimes I say, "Hospice is the best thing that has ever happened to medicine." Obviously, there are things that have had more impact—like understanding germ theory and the use of antibiotics, and, ah, yes, hand washing. Still, it was wonderful to be part of hospice care, a truly amazing gift for patients who face a life-limiting illness and their families.

My reason for sharing these stories is to acquaint readers with this fabulous kind of care:

- Readers in general will, I hope, see the possibilities of the various kinds of care available and not be so afraid of facing chronic or terminal illness.
- Patients will ask their medical and family caregivers for the best care available, palliative care by itself and within hospice when appropriate as early as possible.
- Patients who are terminally ill will be less afraid of the concept of hospice and not see it as giving up but as choosing to live to the fullest with the best quality care available.
- Caregivers will find the stories and the insights helpful in their own life journey.

- Medical personnel will see the kindness and wisdom of offering quality comfort care, able to balance the positives and negatives of working for cure versus providing symptom management and comfort, considering quality of life instead of quantity of time.
- Educators will use these stories to guide physicians, nurses, chaplains, social workers, and others in understanding and using palliative and hospice care.
- Volunteers will be encouraged to spend quality time with patients, assisting caregivers, working in thrift shops, and promoting hospice fundraisers. Hospice was begun by volunteers and is now required to have 5 percent of the operations handled by volunteers.
- Social planners will be able to recognize the huge cost savings possible with the hospice concept and less expensive end-of-life care.
- Readers will learn that some patients actually live longer with hospice than they would have, are more comfortable physically and emotionally, and their families have support and manage more easily, and spend quality time with the patient.

Once more I will repeat these stunning figures: six months of hospice care are available. In 2016 in the United States, 40.5 percent of hospice patients received care for fourteen days or less, about one-third of patients received care for seven days or less instead of the six months—180 days—they could have had. What a tragedy! Please request hospice care when it's appropriate for yourself or someone you love.

Working with dying persons reminds us of our own mortality, encourages us to value the joys of life, and helps us to face ultimate things ourselves. In particular, it is fascinating to see the interplay between the wish for independence, the fear of dependence, and the satisfying ways patients, families, and hospice foster warm and healthy interdependence, learn to say goodbye, and manage grief. It was an honor and a joy to be part of that. Why? The answer is in George Eliot's question: "What do we live for, if it is not to make life less difficult to [*sic*] each other?"[2]

From me to you: You have many good choices for end-of-life care. Read, ask questions, talk to your medical practitioners, ask for help, and accept the help available. Find ways to learn early what you and those you love want at the end of life. Talk with your family, talk to your doctor. Think about it all. Make decisions and complete your advance directives. Take good care of yourself and your loved ones.

—I wish you well, Karen

THINGS I WISH WERE DIFFERENT

- I wish hospice was better understood by patients, caregivers, families, educators, health care professionals, retirement center and skilled nursing facility administrators, and policy makers.
- I wish the pros and the cons of treatment were described fully to patients and family members.
- I wish physicians understood that they can bill for end-of-life discussions.
- I wish patients were referred for palliative care for management of severe symptoms.
- I wish patients were referred to hospice when no more treatment is available or wanted.
- I wish that better training in pain and symptom management, cultures and belief systems, and end-of-life care were available to all health care professionals.
- I wish insurance companies and governmental agencies covered more caregiver needs.
- I wish Medicaid benefits did not vary from state to state.
- I wish quality of life issues were considered, and more patients could avoid the often-debilitating cycle of ER visits, ICU, and hospital admissions.
- I wish palliative care and hospice had a bigger voice.

It's my passion and my goal to help demystify so more patients and caregivers can enjoy this extraordinary comfort care.

Appendix A

*Ways to Make a Limited Life More Pleasant
for the Patient and the Caregiver*

COMMUNICATION

Many communication products are available online; look for "message boards." They use smiley faces, objects, and/or the alphabet to assist with communication.[1] You can create devices yourself; one example is the scrapbook made by the children in the story about Kevin and Annie.

FOOD AND DRINK

Check with the doctor or nurse to be sure the ingredients are alright for the patient.

Nutrition Supplements like Ensure © or Boost ©:

- Some folks are happy drinking them just as they come out of the can.
- Cold, sometimes with ice, is more palatable to many people.
- The challenge is to find ways to make these seem like a treat:

    1. Smoothie or milkshake: add fruit and whiz in the blender.
    2. Hot or cold mocha drink: dissolve one teaspoon of instant coffee in hot water; stir it into the chocolate nutritional drink—cool or heat it. Add mint.

3. Sorbet or sherbet/faux—mix in crushed fruit or coffee and/or chocolate and pour it into a freezer tray; when frozen it's a bit like sorbet or sherbet.

Create a Snack Center

Create a special table and chair to make eating interesting and enjoyable.

1. Serve meals at regular meal times—but don't require patients to eat them then.
2. Put leftover food in the refrigerator in nice dishes; serve it when they are interested.
3. Stock a small refrigerator just for the patient; put in an easy to see and use place.
4. Next to it, place an interesting little table with a pretty tablecloth or placemat.
5. Use plastic dishes and glasses that are colorful, won't break, and can be tossed. Some folks benefit from divided dishes or dishes with a raised elope.
6. Create small portions: finger sandwiches, chunks of several kinds of cheeses, peanut butter on celery sticks on a plate, crackers and cheese, with see-through plastic wrap covering it; ready to eat when your patient is hungry or bored.
7. Small containers of yogurt with fruit; some taste like the old fashioned popsicles.
8. Include (approved) small candy bars and suckers and bags of chips.
9. Portion chips and/or crackers in the size you wish them to have.
10. Include tiny restaurant-sized servings of peanut butter, jam, honey, catsup, and mustard.

Dementia-Friendly Ideas

- In the patient's room or at their snack center, use furniture, dishes, and pictures on the wall that are from the time period that he or she most remembers or identifies with.
- Whole countries, cities, and businesses are showing an awareness of Alzheimer's or dementia patients and providing support and services. For instance: In the City of Bruges, Belgium, participating stores identifying their intention to be of help to dementia sufferers and their families display a knotted handkerchief on their door or in their windows.
- Work with agencies in your community to create awareness.

THE PATIENT'S ENVIRONMENT

Make sure the patient has the appropriate shoes, cane, walker, or wheelchair, and that you have permission from your patient's physician or therapist.

1. Walk with the patient in your neighborhood, a park, playground, church grounds, or schools (stay a safe distance if they wish you to).
2. Take advantage of the patient's "wandering" and you or a friend take him or her for walks.
3. Some assisted living and patient medical facilities create safe walking paths because walking outdoors is good for patients, visiting family and staff.
4. Recliners can replace beds when helpful.
5. Pets are part of some assisted living, convalescent, and hospice facilities; when it's reasonable, get a pet, invite trainers and their service animals, or "foster" pets from a local animal shelter.
6. Some patients with any degree of dementia are frightened or confused by some dramatic TV shows as they believe the events are real and happening currently.
7. TV can be a distraction they do not understand or enjoy.
8. Favorite TV shows can be helpful.
9. News events or stories reported frequently, as on cable news, may be believed to be continuously occurring. This was documented during 9/11: young children and folks with dementia issues thought the planes were continuing to hit the buildings.
10. Dramas can be too emotional, disturbing, and distracting.
11. Favorite and/or calming music is a better choice.
12. In a skilled nursing facility or memory unit, TV and radio usage should be part of the care plan.

SAFETY

There are ways to give a gentle message that means "Stop" in front of an elevator, stairway, or outside a door.[2]

1. Velvet rope attached to attractive metal stanchions/posts, like in a theater.
2. A square of black carpet in front of a door; some interpret it as a hold or a change.
3. Yellow tape, similar to police crime scene tape.
4. Use actual "Stop" signs.

5. Purchase bracelets to identify medical or mental issues. There are many options online.

MANAGING DIFFICULT BEHAVIOR

1. Combative and resistant behavior is sometimes due to not-yet-identified pain or another medical issue. Ask your medical professionals to determine pain and other symptomatic problems (for example, nausea) when choosing treatment or medications.
2. When possible and safe, "play along" with delusions; it's comforting to the patient and is a way to learn more about the patient's history, thinking, and fears.[3]
3. Let the patient choose what time of day to bathe, take a walk, and see visitors.
4. Sometimes just a different word or phrase may help:

    a. "life-limiting" instead of "terminal illness";
    b. "having trouble thinking" instead of "dementia" or "Alzheimer's disease."

Appendix B

Selected Bibliography

Allen, Woody. *Without Feathers*. New York: Ballantine Books, 1976.

Boss, Pauline. *Ambiguous Loss: Learning to Live with Unresolved Grief*. Cambridge, MA: Harvard University Press, 2000.

Bugajski, Ben. "Professor Reflects on Life Work in Hospice Care." *The University Record*, University of Michigan, Lansing, Michigan. September 18, 2017.

Callanan, Maggie, and Patricia Kelley. *Final Gifts: Understanding the Special Awareness, Needs and Communications of the Dying*. New York: Simon and Schuster, 2012.

Carlisle, Patrick. *Unfair and Unbalanced: The Lunatic Magniloquence of Henry E. Panky*. Cranston, RI: Writers' Collective, 2006.

Eliot, George. Chapter 71 in *Middlemarch* [1871]. Boston: Charles E. Lauriat Co., 1908.

Fanestil, John. *Mrs. Hunter's Happy Death: Lessons on Living from People Preparing to Die*. New York: Doubleday, 2006.

Frankl, Viktor. *Man's Search for Meaning* [1946]. Boston: Beacon Press, 2006.

Gawande, Atul. *Being Mortal: Medicine and What Matters in the End*. New York: Picador, 2014.

Geymay, John. *Souls on a Walk: An Enduring Love Story Unbroken by Alzheimer's*. New York: Copernicus Healthcare, 2012.

Gordon, Steve, and Irene Kacandes. *Let's Talk About Death: Asking the Questions that Profoundly Change the Way We Live and Die*. Amherst, NY: Prometheus Books, 2016.

Harris, Maxine. *The Loss that Is Forever: The Lifelong Impact of the Early Death of a Mother or Father*. New York: Plume Books, 1996.

Hospice Foundation of America. *Guide for Recalling and Retelling Your Life Story*. Washington, DC: Hospice Foundation of America, 2001.

Kubler-Ross, Elizabeth. *On Death and Dying*. New York: Macmillan, 1969.

Lear, Norman. *Even This I Get to Experience*. London: Penguin, 2014.

Lewis, C. S. *A Grief Observed*. New York: A Bantam Book/The Seabury Press, 1961.

Mace, Nancy L., and Peter V. Rabins. *The 36-Hour Day*. Ninth edition. Baltimore: Johns Hopkins University Press, 2006.

Mead, Rebecca. "New Ways to Care for People with Dementia." *The New Yorker*. May 5, 2013.

Moody, Raymond. *Life After Life*. Seattle: Mockingbird Books, 1975.

National Hospice and Palliative Care Organization. *2016 Annual Report. Facts and Figures: Hospice Care in America*. Alexandria, VA.

Pabst, Margery, and Rita Goldhammer. *Enrich Your Caregiving Journey*. Andover, MN: Expert Publishing Inc., 2009.

Park, Alice. "Alzheimer's Unlocked." *TIME*. October 25, 2010.

Patterson, Beth S. *The Long Goodbye: When Someone You Love Has Alzheimer's*. New York: Riverhead Books, 2011.

The Regence Foundation. *National Journal* poll of 500 physicians, reported in "Living Well at the End of Life: A National Conversation." February 16, 17, 19, 2011, http://www.syndication.nationaljournal.com/communications/NationalJournalRegenceToplines.pdf.

Ross, Kate. "The Final Act: Lucinda Herring Helps Families Care for Their Dead." *Whidbey Life Magazine*. April 19, 2017.

Russo, Richard, ed. *A Healing Touch: True Stories of Life, Death, and Hospice*. Lanham, MD: Down East Books, an Imprint of Rowman & Littlefield, 2008.

Seneca, Lucius Annaeus (Seneca the Younger) 4 BC–65 AD. http://www.sophia-project.org/uploads/1/3/9/5/13955288/seneca_anger.pdf.

Shacter, Phyllis. *Choosing to Die: A Personal Journey*. Create Space, 2017. See also "Not Here by Choice, TEDx Bellingham.

Sheehy, Gail. *Passages in Caregiving*. New York: G. Merrit Corp., 2010.

Shilts, Randy. *And the Band Played On: Politics, People and the AIDS Epidemic*. New York: St. Martin's Press, 1987. Also 1993 a docudrama by HBO Films, Spelling Productions.

Soloman, Andrew. *The Noonday Demon: An Atlas of Depression*. New York: Simon and Schuster, 2002.

Span, Paula. *When the Time Comes: Families with Aging Parents Share Their Struggles and Solutions*. New York: Springboard Press, 2009.

Stevenson, Adlai E. II. "The Nature of Patriotism." Address to the American Legion Convention, Madison Square Garden, New York City, August 27, 1952.

Sutton, Kate. "Guidelines for Talking with Children about Grief." Posted on eHospice website. http://www.lifecare.com/blog. First published on Transitions LifeCare blog, February 2, 2016.

Tedeschi, Bob. @bobtedeschi "As the End Nears, 'Death Doulas' Ease the Way." STAT e-newsletter, April 7, 2016. http://www.statnews.com/2016/04/07/death-doulas-end-of-life.

Trowbrige, David Daiku. *Enso House: Caring for Each other at the End of Life*. Freeland, WA: Abiding Nowhere Press, 2012.

Ussher, Parick. "Hidden Dementia Grief," quoting Breffni McGuiness. NHPCO, eHospice, Article from Hospice of Ireland, Dublin, Ireland, March 3, 2017.

Volandes, Angelo. *The Conversation: A Revolution Plan for End-of-Life Care*. New York: Bloomsbury, 2015.

Warner, Mark L. *In Search of the Alzheimer's Wanderer*. Workbook. Amazon, 2005.

Weissman, David E., ed. *Fast Fact*. First edition. Milwaukee: Palliative Care Network of Wisconsin.

Whitney, Christie. *Videos for Grieving Children*. Partners in Parenting in Association with Listen 2 Kids Production, 2010–2013.

William, Terry Tempest: *Refuge: An Unnatural History of Family and Place*. New York: Pantheon, 1991.

Wright, Alexi, et al. "Family Perspectives on Aggressive Cancer Care Near the End of Life." *Journal of the American Medical Association* 31 (2016): 284–92.

Appendix C

Suggested Reading

Books and articles written by health care professionals, chaplains, social workers, spouses, children, counselors, journalists, and volunteers.

Appleton, Michael. *Good End: End-of-life Concerns and Conversations about Hospice and Palliative Care*. Tucson, AZ: Hats Off Books, 2005.

Agronin, Marc E. *The Dementia Caregiver: A Guide to Caring for Someone with Alzheimer's Disease and Other Neurogenitive Disorders*. Lanham, MD: Rowman & Littlefield, 2015.

Barr, Niki. *Emotional Well-Being: The Other Half of Treating Cancer*. Seattle: Orion Wellspring, Inc., 2012.

Beecham, Jahnna, and Katie Ortlip. *Living with Dying: The Complete Guide for Caregivers*. New York: Columbia University Press, 2016.

Bell, Karen Whitley. *Living at the End of Life: A Hospice Nurse Addresses the Most Common Questions*. New York: Sterling Publishing, 2010.

Bradley, Rosaline. *A Matter of Life and Death: 60 Voices Share Their Wisdom*. London: Jessica Kingsley Publishers. 2016.

Brooks, Barbara, and Paula M. Siegel. *The Scared Child: Helping Kids Overcome Traumatic Events*. Hoboken, NJ: Wiley, 1996.

Buckingham, Robert, PhD. *Among Friends: Hospice Care for the Person with AIDS*. Buffalo, NY: Prometheus Books, 1992. And multiple groundbreaking earlier works including guides and workbooks on hospice in its early days in the United States and on grief. See also Ben Bugajski's article, "Professor Reflects on Life Work in Hospice Care." *The University Record*, University of Michigan, Lansing, Michigan, September 18, 2017.

Burack-Weiss, Ann, Lynn Sara Lawrence, and Lynne Bamat Mijangos, eds. *Narrative in Social Work Practice: The Power and Possibility of Story*. New York: Columbia University Press, 2017.

Callanan, Maggie, and Patricia Kelley. *Final Gifts: Understanding the Special Needs and Communications of the Dying*. New York: Bantam Books, 1997.

Didion, Joan. *The Year of Magical Thinking*. New York: Alfred A. Knopf, 2005.

Duke, Robert. *Waking up Dying: Caregiving When There Is No Tomorrow*. Bellingham, WA: Good Enough Publishing, 2014.

Green, John. *The Fault in Our Stars*. Boston: Dutton Books, 2012. (Also a film for young adults.)

Heart, Maria Dansing. *The Last Adventure of Life: Sacred Resources for Living and Dying from a Hospice Counselor*. Findhorn, Scotland: Findhorn Press, 2008.

Holford, Karen. *I Miss Grandpa*. Anaheim, CA: Pacific Press Publishing Association, 2004.

Kessler, David. *The Needs of the Dying: A Guide for Bringing Hope, Comfort, and Love to Life's Final Chapter*. New York: Harper Collins, 2007.

Klunder, Kerry. *The Complex Maze Called Hospice Social Work: A Realistic and Light-Hearted Look at the Roles and Techniques of Hospice Social Workers*. Parker, CO: Outskirts Press, 2011.

Lattanzi-Licht, Marcia, Galen W. Miller, and John J. Mahoney. *The Hospice Choice: In Pursuit of a Peaceful Death*. New York: Fireside; The National Hospital Organization in association with Simon and Schuster, 1998.

Lembke, Janet. *Quality of Life: Living Well, Dying Well*. Guilford, CT: Lyons Press, 2003.

Lindner, Eric. *Lessons for Living at the End of Life*. Lanham, MD: Rowman & Littlefield, 2013.

Miller, James E. *The Art of Being a Healing Presence*. Ft. Wayne, IN: Willowgreen, 2001.

Mundy, Michaelene. *Sad Isn't Bad: A Good-Grief Guidebook for Kids Dealing with Loss*. Saint Meinrad, IN: Abbey Press, 1998.

Nuland, Sherwin B. *How We Die: Reflections on Life's Final Chapter*. New York: Vintage, 2006.

Parker, Frances Shani. *Becoming Dead Right: A Hospice Volunteer in Urban Nursing Homes*. Ann Arbor, MI: Loving Healing Press, 2007.

Parry, Joan K. *Social Work Theory and Practice with the Terminally Ill*. Second edition. Binghamton, NY: Haworth Social Work Practice Press, 2000.

Plish, Dana. *The Dying Process—A Hospice Social Worker's Perspective on End-of-Life Care: A Helpful Guide for Coping and Closure during End of Life Care*. North Charleston, SC: Createspace, 2014.

Rabey, Lois, and Steve Rabey. *Lesson for the Living from the Dying: Finding Wisdom in Final Conversations*. Colorado Springs: Bondfire Books, 2013.

Remnick, David. "In the Archives: The Widow's Peak." *The New Yorker*. June 18, 2012.

Schwiebert, Pat, and Chuck Deklyen. *Tear Soup*. Portland, OR: Grief Watch, 2010.

Ubel, Peter A. *Critical Decisions: How You and Your Doctor Can Make the Right Medical Choices Together*. San Francisco, CA: Harper One, 2012.

Wagner, Richard. *The Amateur's Guide to Death and Dying: Enhancing the End of Life*. Austin, TX: The Nazca Plains Corporation. 2012.

Wyatt, Karen. *What Really Matters: Lessons for the Living from the Stories of the Dying*. Silverthorne, CO: Sunroom Studios, 2013.

Appendix D

Glossary, Terms, and Abbreviations

AARP: American Association of Retired Persons, providing information, a magazine, and services to seniors.

ACP: Advanced care planning helps those battling chronic and terminal illnesses know about their options and create appropriate advance directives so they receive the care they want and don't receive the care they don't want.

ACS: American Cancer Society, an organization funding cancer research and providing information and services for cancer patients, their families, the public, and health care communities, and in some areas, transportation to medical treatments and support groups.

ADL: Activities of daily living, including eating, bathing, dressing, toileting, transferring (walking), and continence.

Adult Day Care: Supervised care during the day; often lunch is provided for whole-day stays.

Advance Directives: Documents providing detailed instructions to health care professionals and medical facilities of what will take place only during the time a person is not able to make his or her own decisions. A health care proxy or agent is named to make those decisions when a person is incapacitated. Included is a living will, medical directive or power of attorney for health care, and code status in a hospital setting. POLST and MOLST are sometimes used (see description below). Nonmedical advance directives include a power of attorney for financial decisions and a will or trust naming beneficiaries.

Advocate: Someone who speaks for folks who need representation; also called an ombudsman. See appendix E, "Helpful Websites," for contact information for various ombudsmen.

After-Death Care: All persons may choose the way a body is managed after death, including (1) having a home funeral service (doulas can assist); (2) viewing, a funeral or memorial service prior, then cremation; (3) cremation without viewing, followed by a memorial service; and (4) using a funeral home services. Note: Embalming may have been chosen by the deceased; if not, the family can always choose to not use embalming—it is costly and invasive. Services can be held within a short time if embalming is not used.

ALS: Amyotrophic lateral sclerosis, a progressive neurodegenerative disease affecting nerve cells in the brain, with devastating medical consequences. See also Lou Gehrig's disease.

Alternative Practices: Complementary and alternative medicine.

Alzheimer's: A progressive, degenerative disorder thought to be due to damaged or missing nerve cells; there are behavioral changes due to loss of memory. Thinking and language skills and eventually movement can be affected. A gentle way of describing this phenomena is "having trouble thinking." See also dementia.

Ambiguous Loss: A living person lost to us due to dementia or a soldier missing in action; offers alternating hope and hopelessness that is exhausting and can be debilitating.

Antibiotics/Abx: Medication used to treat bacterial infections.

Apnea: Extended periods when breathing stops during sleep.

Artificial Nutrition and Hydration (ANH): Life-sustaining treatments administered through nasal or abdominal tubes or a vein. When the dying process has begun and the body is shutting down, these treatments may overburden the system and the patient may become uncomfortable. When a patient is near death, often there will not be a feeling of hunger. The website for guidelines for the use of ANH is found in appendix E.

CAM: Complementary and alternative medicine. See also traditional medicine and alternative practices.

Caregiving: About forty million persons provide unpaid caregiving to others—spouses, children, siblings, parents, and friends; approximately 40 percent of them are men.

Celebration of Life: Services can occur before a death occurs with the ill person enjoying it with their family and friends or after death. Locations can be in a home, church, hall, funeral home, or at the graveside—creative celebrations are encouraged.

Chaplain: A person trained to be a spiritual guide, skilled at supporting a person's beliefs.

Cheyne-Stokes Breathing: An abnormal pattern of breathing that may be deeper and/or faster breathing, followed by periods of temporarily stopping breathing or apnea; it can cycle from a few seconds to up to two minutes, and can be an indication of the dying process.

Combative Behavior: Persons acting aggressively (hitting, kicking, refusing meals, etc.), as sometimes happens with persons with Alzheimer's disease or other dementia. Sometimes physical symptoms can exacerbate the behavior—pain, nausea, apnea, hunger, or medication imbalance.

Comfort Care/Palliative Care: All care is intended to provide comfort to the patient; palliation is another word for comfort and is the primary focus of hospice care for terminally ill patients. Palliative care is a relatively new specialty that focuses on management of difficult symptoms (for example, pain, nausea, apnea, anorexia, or edema) of those who are not terminal. All care is palliative (for comfort); not all palliative care is hospice care.

Congestive Heart Failure (CHF): Heart failure characterized by the heart's inability to pump an adequate supply of blood.

COPD: Congestive obstructive pulmonary (or lung) disease. See also emphysema.

Continuing Bonds: A theory about grief focusing on "finding new and different relationships" with the memory of the person who died.

CPR: Cardiopulmonary resuscitation.

Continuity of Care: Quality medical care includes preventative, emergency, attention to health and chronic conditions, and care for the terminally ill.

Cremains: Cremated remains, or what remains after a cremation. These are often kept by family members in an urn of plastic, wood, metal, or stone. There are guidelines in each state about where they can be dispersed.

Cultural Assessment: Basic questions asked to determine a patient's understanding of his or her illness and its causes and possible cures as seen in his or her belief system, values, and practices.

Culture: "Culture is the complete way of a people, learned and integrated into life" (Gottfried Oosterwal, medical anthropologist, deceased; personal communication 1981).

Death Midwife/Death Doula/Spiritual Midwives/Soul Midwives: Persons trained to be with patients, families, caregivers, and friends to assist in their wishes to be involved in the death and after-death care of individuals. Certification is available.

DNACPR: Do not attempt CPR.

DNI: Do not intubate.

DNR: Do not resuscitate.

Death and Dying Movement: Begun in the United States by Elizabeth Kubler-Ross, Swiss psychiatrist. She taught health care professionals about end-of-life care, urging that family members be involved.

Dementia: Having trouble thinking. See also Alzheimer's disease.

Diagnosis/Dx: The act of determining a disease by its signs and symptoms.

Directive to Physicians: This is a legal document that describes your wishes about the level of medical treatment you prefer when (1) you are determined to be terminally ill, or (2) have an irreversible condition in which you are unable to make decisions for yourself and are expected to die without life-sustaining procedures. Also called a "Living Will." Most states have websites which provide the appropriate documents. It is not in effect if you are pregnant. It may be revoked at any time. It is one of the "advance directives" folks are urged to complete.

Disenfranchised Grief: Grief that is not acknowledged or understood by society as significant. Examples include the grief of a person with dementia who recognizes there are problems thinking but cannot understand or describe them; also grief from experiencing miscarriage, placing a child for adoption, death or loss of a pet, many moves (e.g., military families).

Doula (Death Doula)/Death Midwife: A person trained to assist patients and families experience death at home. Doulas also help with funerals and burials.

Edema: Excessive accumulation of fluid in the tissues.

Emphysema: A disease in which the lungs become impaired and breathing is difficult. See also COPD.

End-of-Life Choices and Decisions: Each person is encouraged to understand the choices he or she has when he or she is near the end of his or her life; in order to have his or her choices honored, it is vital that each person learn about the choices and create documents that describe those choices and the agents he or she wishes to help when he or she cannot make decisions for him- or herself. These documents are called advance directives. Good information about the choices and the documents are available on the internet and through legal representatives.

End-Stage Disease: Health care professionals use this term when there is no cure available. Hospices use Medicare guidelines to determine the end stage for each illness.

Ethnicity: A sense of peoplehood, usually including geographic location, language, belief system, cultural practices, and traditions. Contrast with race, a social construct.

Funeral: A service usually in a funeral home or with the guidance of a funeral home and held in a church or hall, or at the graveside. The deceased may be in an open or closed casket; the casket may also remain in a side viewing room at the request of the family. Ashes may be in an urn. See also celebration of life for further options.

Green Burial: Burial in which there is no embalming and the body is placed in a community cemetery or a natural burial ground. The film "A Will for the Woods" tells the story of one family who choose green burial.

Grief: Natural and normal reaction to an abnormal situation, like the loss of a loved one, friend, family member, or even pets; also the loss a job, your home, or other significant change. There are many theories and descriptions of processing grief, such as the very basic and limited Five Stages of Kubler-

Ross. See also ambiguous loss, disenfranchised grief, and hidden dementia grief.

Grieving: Moving through the reactions and feelings of loss.

Guest Book: Small lined book for guests to sign their names and make comments if they wish when attending a funeral, life celebration, graveside service, or green burial.

Having Trouble Thinking: A term used to describe aspects of dementia and Alzheimer's disease.

Hidden Dementia Grief: The dementia patient's grief at recognizing that he or she does not remember, cannot place or recognize faces and names, and has losses he or she can't even describe or articulate.

Home Health Aide: A trained and certified health care worker usually offering physical care.

Hospice: "Hospice is a holistic, team-oriented program of care which seeks to treat and comfort terminally ill patients and their families at home or in a home-like setting" (definition from the National Hospice Organization). Originally these were places for travelers or the ill to rest and be cared for and the word comes from the root for "hospitality" including both host and guest. Now the term is used for organizations providing end-of-life care, in a person's home, a place they call home, or a hospice house.

Hospice Advocate: Every one who has compassion for and helps to education about end-of-life issues.

Kids' Group: Support groups offered to children by mental health care professionals to help manage the questions, fears, and concerns relating to important life events or changes.

Kubler-Ross, Elizabeth: Swiss psychiatrist, well known for her studies and writings about death and dying, focusing on five basic reactions: shock and/or denial, anger, bargaining, depression, and acceptance. It is not expected that each person feels each of these reactions or experiences them in any particular order.

LGBTIQ: Lesbian/gay/bisexual/transgender or transsexual/intersexual/queer orientation.

Life-Limiting Illness: Terminal illness. Life expectancy of six months or less.

Life Review: Suggestions for talking with patients and family members about special experiences in their lives using photos, stories, and memories to identify important and meaningful people and places and remember their personal contributions.

Life-Sustaining Procedures: Artificial means of keeping persons alive, hydrated, and fed, including intubation (mechanical ventilation), blood transfusions, and feed tubes. It is the constitutional right of each individual to refuse treatment of any kind.

Living Will: See advance directives, Directive to Physician.

Logotherapy: Treatment perspective helping people remember things that gave/gives their lives meaning. Originated by Viktor Frankl, Austrian psychiatrist and Holocaust survivor.

Lou Gehrig's Disease: See ALS.

Medical Examiner: A person qualified and assigned to make an official pronouncement of death. Some other medical personnel are allowed by law to make the pronouncement.

Memorial Services: Remembrance services held without the presence of the deceased; can be held days, weeks, or months after a death. Location is at the discretion of the family and friends.

Metastasis: An infection or cancer spreading beyond the original site.

NDE: Near-death experiences. Multiple sensations may include feelings of detachment, peace, and so forth.

Nonreimbursable: No payment required; sometimes called "charity" or "not-for-profit."

Nutrition Supplements: Over-the-counter products that provide safe nutrition for persons who are not getting a balanced diet due to intake restrictions or preferences. See appendix A for ways to make them more palatable. Check first with physician or nurse.

OBE: Out of body experiences, usually experienced with extreme mental or physical trauma.

Okay: Alright. This item is included here because end-of-life issues are associated with two meanings: (1) things are acceptable, as in "death is a natural process and the time comes for each person to accept that it's happening and that it's normal" (see the story of Viola) and (2) it does not feel alright to be facing the end of one's existence (see Annie's story).

Ombudsman: Someone who speaks for folks who need representation; also called an advocate. See appendix E, "Helpful Websites," for contact information for various ombudsmen.

Options for Care: Treatment for cure, "watchful waiting," and palliative (comfort care) are available through the palliative care specialty and through hospice organizations.

Pain Issues: The focus of palliative/comfort care is to manage pain and other symptoms.

Pain Scale: Number scales are used (0 [no pain] through 10 [the worst you can imagine]); often drawings of faces are used, showing differing degrees of discomfort. Check the internet for various scales and other devices to help the patient express his or her feelings and needs.

Palliative/Comfort Care: Treatment to manage symptoms causing discomfort is always a part of patient care and can be chosen as the focus when no treatment or cure is available or desired, as in hospice care. All care is intended to provide comfort to the patient; palliation is another word for comfort and is the primary focus of hospice care for terminally ill patients.

Palliative care is a relatively new specialty that focuses on management of difficult symptoms (for example, pain, nausea, apnea, anorexia, or edema) of those who are not terminal. All care is palliative (for comfort); not all palliative care is hospice care.

PO: Represents *per os*; means given by mouth.

POLST/MOLST: Physician (or medical) orders for life-sustaining treatment forms used to document decisions made with the patient's physician to indicate treatments he or she wants and those he or she does not want. Other health care workers (for example, nurses, social workers, and chaplains) may help the patient and family understand the form and the choices. These forms should be prominently displayed in the patient's room so that EMTs and other workers will be able to follow the patient's wishes about his or her care.

Powers of Attorney: Forms designating persons who are to take responsibility at the event of or during the time of the patient being unable to make decisions.

PRN: Abbreviation for *pro re nata*; means as the occasion arises or when necessary.

Quality of Life: A good standard of physical and mental health and relationships.

Race: Identification of persons based on the supposed physical differences in skin color and looks. There is no scientific basis for this category and it is rejected on a scientific basis; race is a social construct. Contrast with ethnicity.

Rare Caregivers: The National Alliance for Caregiving and Global Genes has released a report on rare diseases in America. They give an estimate of seven hundred rare diseases, with cystic fibrosis leading the way in numbers affected. Caregivers are often stressed financially and emotionally; sometime they even say they need to train health care workers in the care of their patients. Palliative and hospice care will need to continue to learn about these diseases to adequately and appropriately help these patients and caregivers.

Refusing Treatment: Patients have a constitutional right to refuse treatment, including nutrition and hydration.

Respite: Time away from patient responsibilities; a rest for the caregiver.

Sepsis: Infection spreading throughout the system. This can become serious quickly.

Snack Center for Patients: See appendix A.

Sociology: The study of how people behave as they live in groups and develop a sense of self.

Spiritual or Soul Midwives: Persons trained to be with patient, families, caregivers, and friends to assist in their wishes to be involved in the death and after-death care of individuals. See also doula (death doula)/death midwife.

Stat: From *statum*; meaning right away.

Suicide: A person actively or passively causes his or her own death.

Syndrome: A group of symptoms indicating a certain disease or condition.

Terminal: Life-limiting. Used when patients are not expected to live more than six months.

Titrate: To gradually adjust the dose of a medication to determine the most effective dose.

Traditional Medicine: Practices and treatments that come from the culture of the patient.

Treatment/Tx: Providing medical diagnosis and care.

VSED: Voluntarily stopping eating and drinking. Some patients with illnesses that often result in dementia, like Alzheimer's, choose to voluntarily stop eating and drinking. The decision must be made while the patient is lucid and requires extensive legal advice and medical guidance. Hospice organizations will need to develop guidelines about working with VSED patients and their caregivers when the person is truly near death.

Appendix E

Helpful Websites

Advance Care Planners, accessed December 25, 2017, http://www.medicare.gov/coverage/advance-care-planning.html

Advanced Directives from National Hospice and Palliative Care Organization, accessed December 25, 2017, http://www.caringinfo.org/i4a/pages/index.cfm?pageid=3277.

Advanced Directives: check in your state. For example, accessed December 25, 2017, https://www.endoflifewa.org.

Alzheimer's Organization, accessed December 25, 2017, www.alz.org. For families, accessed December 25, 2017, www.helpforalzheimersfamilies.com.

American Cancer Society, accessed December 25, 2017, www.cancer.org. Information about specific cancers, connection to survivors, and fundraising for cancer research. In some areas there are support groups, transportation to treatment, and volunteering.

American Lung Association (for example, cancer, COPD), accessed December 25, 2017, www.lung.org.

Cancer.Net (see especially the section on "Hospice Care"), accessed December 25, 2017, https://www.cancer.net/navigating-cancer-care/advanced-cancer/hospice-care.

Caregiver's Guide re: Dementia Behaviors, accessed December 25, 2017, www.caregiver.org/caregivers-guide-understanding-dementia-behaviors.

Caregiver Stress, accessed December 25, 2017, www.caregiverstress.com.

Caregiving, accessed December 25, 2017, www.aarp.org/caregiving.

Caregiving, Asian American and Pacific Islander Communities, accessed December 25, 2017, www.aarp.org/aapi.

Caregiving, from the National Hospice and Palliative Care Organization (NHPCO) (see "The Dying Process—A Guide for Family Caregivers"), accessed December 17, 2017, http://www.caringinfo.org/files/public/brochures/UnderstandingtheDyingProces.pdf.

Caring Village 2017, "Caregiving 101 Checklist," accessed December 25, 2017, https://www.caringvillage.com/wp-content/uploads/2017/02/caregiving101_checklist.pdf.

Courageous Parents Network (includes video library), accessed December 25, 2017, www.courageousparentsnetwork.org.

Crossings: Caring for Our Own at Death, accessed December 25, 2017, http://crossings.net/resources.html.

Death Café (regular meetings of folks who want to discuss all aspects of death and dying, worldwide sites), accessed December 25, 2017, http://deathcafe.com/.

End of Life/Washington/Instructions, Advance Documents (downloadable): check your state information. See your attorney, accessed December 13, 2017, http://www.endoflife/wa. Instructions, documents, confer with your health care professional, notarize.

Facebook after Death, accessed December 25, 2017, www.mashable.com/2013/02/13/facebook-after-death.

Family Caregiver Alliance, facts and tip sheets available in English, Spanish, Chinese, Korean, and Vietnamese; includes legal, LGBT, etc., accessed December 25, 2017, https://www.caregiver.org/.

Final Passage, accessed December, 25, 2017, www.finalpassages.org.

Funeral Guide/World-Wide (see THANOS, the world organization of funeral directors, with information about embalming options, transportation, and links to related sites), accessed December 27, 2017, http://thanos.org/en/page/home/.

Goulet, John, "The Four Feeling Groups," accessed December 25, 2017, http://www.johngouletmft.com/The_Four_Feeling_Groups.pdf.

Green Burial, for example, White Eagle Natural Burial Ground, Goldendale, WA 98620, accessed December 26, 2017, http://naturalburialground.org/.

Grief and Bereavement, General Guidelines, National Institutes of Health, U.S. National Library of Medicine, accessed December 13, 2017, https://medlineplus.gov/bereavement.html.

Health Information, accessed December 25, 2017, www.nia.nih.gov.

Home Funerals: many online resources; use a search engine to see those in your area.

Home Instead Senior Care, a network to help you search for adult home care, accessed December 13, 2017, www.HomeInstead.com/HomeCare.

Home Safety Guidelines, Caregiver Center, accessed December 25, 2017, https://www.alz.org.

Hospice Compare Websites, Centers for Medicare Services, released August 17, 2017, accessed December 25, 2017, https://www.medicare.gov/hospice.

Hospice Foundation of America; many publications and other help. Washington: HFA, accessed December 13, 2017, http://hospicefoundation.org/.

Hospice Patient's Bill of Rights, enhanced by new Medicare rule, accessed December 25, 2017, http://www.medicareadvocacy.org/hospice-patients-rights-enhanced-by-new-medicare-rule.

How to Have Difficult Conversations, for example, "Let's Talk about Death & Dying," Lesley Carter, illustrated by Bagi Froden, accessed December 25, 2017, accessed December 25, 2017, http://www.eolc.co.uk/uploads/talking_about_death_booklet_final_version.pdf.

Muscular Dystrophy Association 2017, Look for Signs and Symptoms, States, and More, accessed December 25, 2017, https://www.mda.org/disease/amyotrophic-lateral-sclerosis.

Myths: The Common Myths about Hospice, Angela Morrow, March 1, 2017, accessed December 26, 2017, https://www.verywell.com/hospice-myths-1132617.

National Alliance for Caregiving and AARP, accessed December 13, 2017, www.caregiving.org/caregiving2015.

National Aphasia Society, accessed December 26, 2017, www.aphasia.org.

National Cancer Institute, at the National Institutes of Health, see especially "Advanced Cancer," accessed December 13, 2017, https://www.cancer.gov/about-cancer/advanced-cancer and https://www.cancer.gov/about-cancer/advanced-cancer/care-choices/care-fact-sheet.

National Home Funeral Alliance, accessed December 25, 2017, www.homefuneralalliance.org.

National Hospice and Palliative Care (NHPCO), accessed December 13, 2017, www.nhpco.org.

National Hospice and Palliative Care (NHPCO), 2016 Facts and Figures, accessed December 26, 2017, http://www.nhpco.org/sites/default/files/public/Statistics_Research/2016_Facts_Figures.pdf.

National Prison Hospice Association (NPHA), accessed December 26, 2017, https://npha.org/.

Palliative Care (see National Hospice and Palliative Care [NHPCO]).

Palliative Care Network of Wisconsin, Fast Facts, accessed December 26, 2017, https://www.mypcnow.org.

Preferences: discover, share, and store end-of-life preferences; website and app, accessed December 26, 2017, https://www.joincake.com/welcome/.

Translation Help: Google the country or language. Some communities have assistance; talk to the social worker at your local hospital.

Voluntarily Stopping Eating and Drinking (VSED). See Phyllis Shacter's website for her TEDx/Bellingham talk describing her husband's and her decision, titled "Not Here by Choice," and her book *Choosing To Die: A Personal Story: Elective Death by Voluntarily Stopping Eating and Drinking (VSED) in the Face of Degenerative Disease* (CreateSpace, 2017).

The author offers these sites as information only and does not endorse them.

Appendix F

Films that May Help Discussions of End-of-Life Issues

And the Band Played On. A look at the history of the HIV/AIDS crisis, movement, and research. Drama with fact-based material. Serious, difficult material—medically and culturally. Based on Randy Shilts's 1983 book of the same name.

Angels in America. HBO miniseries. Intense, bawdy, R-rated. Directed by Mike Nichols, based on Tony Kushner's play. Wide-ranging stories involving politics. Set in the mid-1980s, the series revolves around six New Yorkers whose lives intersect in a changing political and cultural climate.

Beaches. Longtime friends, played by Bette Midler and Barbara Hershey, manage many life challenges and examine and enrich their friendship in the face of death.

Bucket List. Morgan Freeman and Jack Nicholson's characters share a hospital room and both have a terminal diagnosis. They make choices about friendship and how to best spend their last few weeks or months. Directed by Rob Reiner.

Life as a House. The story of an architect who decides to build a house after he receives a terminal diagnosis, hoping to heal the relationship with his son.

Me Before You. Adapted from the bestselling novel by Jo Jo Moyes, *Me Before You.* A young English woman is hired to care for a young, wealthy, paralyzed young man.

Memorial Day. A grandfather shares some memories of war with his grandson after the grandson finds his footlocker. Starring James Cromwell.

Miss You Already. Beautiful story of a longtime friendship; one friend becomes terminally ill and goes into care at a hospice house. Starring Drew Barrymore and Toni Collette.

My Life. Michael Keaton portrays a young married man with kidney cancer who, when told he and his wife will have a child, makes videos of his life as teaching tools for his son. They use hospice at home.

Step Mom. This story faces the challenges of a second marriage and the first mom's illness and impending death. Starring Susan Sarandon, Ed Harris, and Julia Roberts.

Story Crops. PBS books, films, foundation. "Listening is an act of love" is their motto.

Tuesdays with Morrie. Reenactment of Mitch Albom's book about his friendship with his dying mentor. Featuring Hank Azaria and Jack Lemon.

A Will for the Woods. Tells the story of Clark Wang choosing green burial. Contemplative.

To assist children, also see ***Partners in Parenting, DVDs for Kids***.

Appendix G

The Differences between Home Health Care,
Palliative Care, and Hospice

Home Health Services

- Medical personnel coming to your home may be offered for a limited time when the patient is released from a hospital stay due to illness or surgery if the expectation is that the patient will be improve and not need the care to continue. A minimum number of days in the hospital may be required.
- Medical personnel may provide care in a patient's home after an illness or injury assisting the patient in learning how to manage their illness, medications, or oxygen, sometimes providing exercises to get stronger or prevent falls. These services may be offered on discharge from the hospital or nursing home, occasionally being offered from a provider office if the need is identified.

Palliative Care

- Palliative care is specialized medical care for people living with serious illness, treating pain and distressing symptoms (e.g., nausea, difficulty sleeping, poor appetite, breathing difficulties) and the stress of the illness. The interdisciplinary team focuses on quality of life, and can help patients decide what care they may or or may not want in the future. They may also help determine when it's time for hospice and help with with that transition.

- Services may be provided in a hospital or where the patient lives, and may be paid for by the patient's insurance plan and/or by Medicare, Medicaid, or Veteran's Benefits.

Hospice Care

- Comfort care when no curative care is available or desired is provided to terminally ill patients, provided by a skilled end-of-life team, offering symptom management and assistance with preparation for death and continuing care during the dying process.
- Services may be provided wherever the paitent lives, and are a benefit of Medicare, Medicaid, Veteran's Benefits, and many private insurances.
- Caregivers and other family members are included in support and care and will continue to be cared for after the death of a loved one, including in support groups.

In small communities, sometimes the same agency offers all three types of service.

Notes

INTRODUCTION

1. Druv Khullar, "We're Bad at Death, Can We Talk?" *New York Times* Op Ed, May 10, 2017.

2. "History of Hospice Care," National Hospice and Palliative Care Organization (NHPCO), September 16, 2015, accessed December 18, 2017, https://www.nhpco.org/history-hospice-care.

3. "Annual Report," National Hospice and Palliative Care Organization (NHPCO), 2016, accessed December 18, 2017, https://www.nhpco.org/sites/default/files/public/governance/Annual_Report_2016.pdf/.

4. David E. Weissman, ed., *Fast Fact*, first edition. (Milwaukee: Palliative Care Network of Wisconsin).

5. Some volunteer groups provide a home for terminally ill patients, using community hospices and other services as needed. One example is in Freeland, Washington, described by David Daiku Trowbridge in his book *Enso House: Caring for Each Other at the End of Life* (Freeland, WA: Abiding Nowhere Press), accessed December 18, 2017, https://jet.com/product/Enso-HouseCaring-for-Each-Other-at-the-End-of-Life/3af6be714d444b4eb38846fe50876a95. There are similar facilities in Tennessee and elsewhere.

6. Alexi Wright, "Family Perspectives on Aggressive Cancer Care Near the End of Life," *Journal of the American Medical Association* 315, no. 3 (2016): 284–92.

7. See Trowbridge, *Enso House.*

8. Health Leaders Media News, "Palliative Care Benefits for Patients Validated," University of Pittsburgh Schools of Medicine and the *Journal of the American Medical Association,* November 23, 2016.

9. Patients in care facilities and their caregivers, including facility medical personnel, may also request a referral to hospice.

10. *Facts and Figures: Hospice Care in America* (National Hospice and Palliative Care Organization [NHPCO], 2017), 3.

1. FIRST VISITS BY THE SOCIAL WORKER

1. Medicare requires that a social worker be on the hospice team and do an assessment within the first five days after the patient chooses hospice care. The decision about how often the social worker visits or phones the patient is made by each hospice organization.

2. C. S. Lewis, *A Grief Observed* (New York: A Bantam Book, The Seabury Press, 1961).

3. Adlai E. Stephenson II, "The Nature of Patriotism," speech given in Madison Square Garden, New York, address to the American Legion Convention, August 27, 1952.

4. Michael H. Levy reports that 65 to 85 percent of those with advanced cancer will have some pain. See "Pharmacologic Treatment of Cancer Pain," *New England Journal of Medicine*, October 10, 1996.

2. HOSPICE CARE AT HOME

1. National Hospice and Palliative Care Organization, *2016 Annual Report: Facts and Figures: Hospice Care in America*, accessed December 18, 2017, https://www.nhpco.org/sites/default/files/public/governance/Annual_Report_2016.pdf/.

2. See the National Aphasia Society website, accessed December 18, 2017, https://www.aphasia.org/.

3. Elizabeth Kubler-Ross, *On Death and Dying* (New York: Macmillan, 1969).

4. Hugh Lofting, 1967. Screenwriter for the film *Dr. Doolittle*. He wrote the original book as well.

5. Terry Tempest Williams, *Refuge: An Unnatural History of Family and Place* (New York: Pantheon, 1991).

6. The phrase "kick the bucket" was used in 1785 this way: "a Great Man, in his querulous twilight years, who doesn't want to go gently into that black black night . . . wants to cut loose, dance on the razor's edge, pry the lid off his bucket." Patrick Carlisle, *Unfair & Unbalanced: The Lunatic Magniloquence of Henry E. Pankey* (Winnipeg, Manitoba: The Writers' Collective, 2006).

7. Muscular Dystrophy Association, "Stages of ALS," 2017, accessed December 18, 2017, https://www.mda.org.

8. TERI: Social Security's program for resources for the terminally ill based on disability benefits, accessed December 17, 2017, https://www.disabilitysecrets.com/resources/disability/social-security-disability-benefits-terminal-i.

9. "National Hospice and Palliative Care Organization: Commentary and Position Statement on Artificial Nutrition and Hydration, Offers Guidelines for Health Care Professionals, Patients, and Family Members," 2010, accessed December 23, 2017, http://www.nhpco.org/sites/default/files/public/ANH_Statement_Commentary.pdf/.

10. Hospices use Medicare guidelines to determine the "end stage" of an illness or disease; still, the determination of "stage" can be very subjective. See the Alzheimer's Association and WebMD websites.

11. John Geymay, *Souls on a Walk: An Enduring Love Story Unbroken by Alzheimers* (New York: Copernicus Healthcare, 2012).

12. Mark L. Warner, *In Search of the Alzheimer's Wanderer: A Workbook* (Amazon, 2012).

13. Nancy L. Mace and Peter V. Rabins, *The 36-hour Day*, ninth edition (Baltimore, MD: Johns Hopkins University Press, 2006).

14. Beth S. Patterson, *The Long Goodbye: When Someone You Love has Alzheimer's* (New York: Riverhead Books, 2011).

15. Pauline Boss, *Ambiguous Loss: Learning to Live with Unresolved Grief* (Cambridge, MA: Harvard University Press, 2000).

16. Patrick Ussher, "Hidden Dementia Grief," quoting Breffni McGuiness (eHospice NHPCO, Article from Hospice of Ireland, Dublin, Ireland, March 3, 2017).

17. Rebecca Mead, "New Ways to Care for People with Dementia," *The New Yorker*, May 5, 2013.

18. Help for Alzheimer's Families website, accessed December 17, 2017, https://www.helpforalzheimersfamilies.com/.

19. *2016 Alzheimer's Disease Association Facts and Figures*, accessed December 17, 2017, https://www.ncbi.nlm.nih.gov/pubmed/27570871/.

20. Alice Park, "Alzheimer's Unlocked," *TIME*, October 25, 2010, accessed December 17, 2017, https://www.amazon.com/Souls-Walk-Enduring-Unbroken-Alzheimers/dp/1938218124.

3. CARING FOR THE CAREGIVER

1. National Alliance for Caregiving and AARP, "Caregiving in the U.S. 2015," accessed December 17, 2017, http://www.caregiving.org/caregiving2015/.

2. Steve Gordon and Irene Kacandes, *Talking about Dying* (Amherst: Prometheus, 2015), 79, 80, 83.

3. Gail Sheehy, *Passages in Caregiving* (New York: G. Merritt Corp, 2010). Sheehy's *Passages* (1976) made her a household name at least for women. She's also written about midlife, menopause, and men's passages.

4. Paula Span, *When the Time Comes: Families with Aging Parents Share Their Struggles and Solutions* (New York: Springboard Press, 2009).

5. Ellen Goodman, the Conversation Project, accessed December 24, 2017, https://theconversationproject.org/.

6. http://www.caregiving.org/wp-content/uploads/2017/11/RAISE_Family_Caregiver_bill_letter.pdf.

7. Rare Disease Caregiving in America. February 2018. A national studying providing information from a partnership of The National Alliance for Caregiving and Global Genes. info@caregiving.org.

8. Margery Pabst and Rita Goldhammer, *Enrich Your Caregiving Journey* (Dudley, England: Expert Publishing Inc., 2009).

4. HOSPICE IN A PLACE YOU CALL HOME

1. Information about local community living choices, seek out the Area Aging on Aging Organization in your state or county, Aging and Disability Services, Federal or County Department of Human Services, and Aging and Long-Term Support Administration, accessed December 17, 2017, https://www.dshs.wa.gov/altsa.

2. Two exquisite examples are found on south Whidbey Island, Washington: (1) Hearts and Hammers, one day a year (and for emergencies) assistance with yard work and home repairs, accessed December 24, 2017, www.heartsandhammers.com/, and (2) South Whidbey at Home, a nonprofit organization, membership-based for age fifty-five and older, "providing access to a variety of professional services, volunteer assistance, and social activities, including when feasible, transportation to medical appointments and grocery shopping." Accessed December 24, 2017, http://swathome.clubexpress.com/.

3. Creative choices, including college campuses, accessed December 17, 2017, http://marks-thomas.com/2016/03/intergenerational-housing-/, and accessed December 17, 2017, http://www.rclco.com/advisory-seniors-housing-innovative-intergenerational-projects.

4. Choices of condos, apartments, homes, managed by the owners, common areas of gardens, community house, and recreational areas. For example, accessed December 17, 2017, https://www.intergenerational-cohousing-for-all-ages.html.

5. One example of women sharing homes, accessed, December 17, 2017, https://www.aarp.org/home-family/your-home/info-05-2013/older-women-roommates-house-sharing.html.

6. Haley Sweetland Edwards, "Dignity, Death and America's Crisis in Elder Care," *TIME*, November 27 through December 4, 2017. A caution is offered to persons choosing SNFs describing that 90 percent of long-term care facilities ask residents to sign a "pre-dispute binding arbitration agreement," giving up Seventh Amendment rights to trial by jury when there is a dispute about care. Some groups are fighting this requirement, but in mid-2017 there was an administration proposal that will allow nursing homes to require that type of agreement and be allowed to turn away applicants who would not sign. The American Health Care Association (AHCA) representing long-term care facilities is involved and presently the outcome is uncertain. This is being challenged by many, including AARP representatives. Families can request help from the ombudsmen available through each state who advocate for patients when there are disputes. Families are limited in the facilities available to them due to cost, location, and availability, and may not know of the arbitration concerns. See "AHCA Sues to Enjoin Prohibition on Binding Arbitration," Health Care Law Today, Foley & Lardner LLP, updated October 10, 2016 by Christopher J. Donovan, Heidi Sorensen, and Matthew Jassak, https://www.healthcarelawtoday.com/2016/10/20/ahca-sues-to-enjoin-prohibition-on-binding-arbitration/. Hospital or SNF social workers can assist patients and families understand and manage financial complications in long-term care facilities.

7. Larry Lipman and Dana E. Neuts, "Where Long-Term Care Works," *AARP Bulletin/ Real Possibilities*, September 2017, p. 38. The Northwest Regional Council provides many services, including tribal outreach, case management, Medicaid transportation, kinship caregiver services, and family caregiver support. Accessed December 17, 2017, http://www.nwrcwa. org/aging-disability-resourcessenior-info-assistance-programs/.

8. That response was exactly what James, the Alzheimer's patient discussed in chapter 3, said when asked about his birthday. Fascinating coincidence, and true.

9. Norman Lear, *Memoir: Even This I Get to Experience* (London: Penguin, 2014).

5. FINDING MEANING

1. Viktor Frankl, *Man's Search for Meaning* (1946; Boston: Beacon Press, 2006).

2. Ben Bugajski, "Professor Reflects on Life Work in Hospice Care," *The University Record* (Lansing: University of Michigan, 2017). This article describes the work of Robert Buckingham, PhD, public health, one of the founding fathers of hospice in America.

3. "Guide for Recalling and Retelling Your Life Story," Hospice Foundation of America, 2001, accessed December 17, 2017, https://hospicefoundation.org/HFA-Products/Guide-for-Recalling-and-Retelling-Your-Life-Story/.

4. Estimates of the number of casualties/deaths range from 4,000 to 6,000, many less than the 20,000 some expected; accessed December 17, 2017, https://fivethirtyeight.com/features/the-challenge-of-counting-d-days-dead/.

5. One of the programs created by Franklin Roosevelt, enlisting unemployed young men in "a peacetime army . . . to battle erosion and destruction of the nation's natural resources," planting trees, building fire towers, forest improvement, disease and insect control, building campgrounds, and more. Accessed December 17, 2017, www.ushistory.com/pages/h1586.

6. John Fanestil, *Mrs. Hunter's Happy Death: Lessons on Living from People Preparing to Die* (New York: Doubleday, 2006).

6. DRAMATIC CHALLENGES

1. Nathan Fairman, Katherine Morrison, Kathy Ligon, Richard Nelesen, and Scott Irwin, "A Retrospective Case Series of Completed Suicides in Hospice (407-B)," *Journal of Pain and Symptom Management* 43, no. 2 (February 2012): 386–87. In their study, men were more likely to complete a suicide attempt, and the choice of weapon was usually a gun; sometimes mental

illness or disability were also factors. Accessed December 24, 2017, http://www.jpsmjournal.com/article/S0885-3924(11)00692-0/fulltext.

2. Kevin Caruso, "Media Guidelines for Suicide Reporting," accessed December 24, 2017, www.suicide.org/media-guidelines-for-suicide.html.

3. John Goulet, "The Four Feeling Groups," accessed December 17, 2017, http://www.johngouletmft.com/The_Four_Feeling_Groups.pdf.

4. "Gun ownership is an ethical, safety concern. Those aged 65 and older now have the highest rate of gun ownership in America, and they also have a high prevalence of depression and suicide. Dementia can add additional layers of risk." Ellen M. Pinholt, Joshua D. Mitchell, Jane H. Butler, and Harjinder Dumar, "'Is There a Gun in the Home?' Assessing the Risks of Gun Ownership in Older Adults," *Journal of American Geriatric Society* (June 4, 2014), accessed December 17, 2017, http://www.medicaldaily.com/gun-ownership-and-elderly-people-over-65-have-highest-rates-ownership-and-dementia-286296.

5. Andrew Solomon, *The Noonday Demon: An Atlas of Depression* (Woodland Park, CO: Touchstone, 2002).

7. SOCIAL ISOLATION

1. Lesbian, gay, bisexual, transsexual, intersexual, queer describes not biological but sexual orientation.

2. National Prison Hospice Association (NPHA), https://npha.org/.

3. "Lucius Annaeus Seneca, Seneca the Younger. 4 BC–65 AD," accessed December 9, 2017, http://www.sophia-project.org/uploads/1/3/9/5/13955288/seneca_anger.pdf.

4. The HIV+ (human immunodeficiency virus) can develop into acquired immunodeficiency syndrome or AIDS.

5. Companies gave patients an agreed-upon amount of cash for their current living expenses and enough for a funeral and the patient would sign for the company to be the beneficiary upon their death.

6. Randy Shilts, *And the Band Played On: Politics, People and the AIDS Epidemic*, 1987. A docudrama was made in 1993 by HBO and Spelling Productions. Both the book and the film provide a good overview of the people infected and affected and the international political influences within the medical world of this new epidemic.

8. SAYING GOODBYE

1. Ashley Benham, a death midwife, writes that "the word 'doula' comes from ancient Greek and is now often used to refer to a woman who helps other women." Doulas help with childbirth and the "meaning is easily transferred for us in death and dying." See her website, accessed December 24, 2017, https://www.asacredpassing.com/wp/wp-content/uploads/2015/02/A-Sacred-Passing-brochure.pdf.

2. Heather Plett, Heather, "What It Really Means to Hold Space for Someone," March 11, 2015, accessed 17 December 17, 2017, http://upliftconnect.com/hold-space/.

3. "The Supreme Court has held that adults have the right to personal autonomy in matters relating to their own medical care." Accessed December 17, 2017, https://www.justia.com/constitutional-law/docs/privacy-rights.html.

4. POLST forms may also be used for terminally ill or frail patients. The acronym stands for "physician orders for life-sustaining treatment" and refers to portable guidelines indicating medical treatment agreed upon by the patient and physician. The physician keeps a copy, and a copy is available for the patient to keep with him or her. See the National POLST Paradigm website, accessed December 24, 2017, http://polst.org/. You can find information about each state's current program; sometimes the name is slightly altered (for example, MOLST).

5. Damage to the body of a frail and/or elderly person can include broken ribs and sometimes paralysis, and he or she may require life support and be cared for in an ICU. When that happens, there will be more decisions that need to be made. Only a small 1 percent of persons who are resuscitated with CPR have a full and meaningful life after that procedure. A good resource for an overview of studies about survival after CPR can be found at http://kokuamau. org/cardiopulmonary-resuscitation-cpr/.

6. Kate Sutton, February 2, 2016, posted on eHospice website, http://www.ehospice.com and first published on the Transitions LifeCare blog https://transitionslifecare.org/blog/.

7. In English influenced by Tagalog, ma'am is a contraction of madam, which sounds to Americans like "mom."

8. Woody Allen, *Without Feathers* (New York: Ballantine Books, 1976).

9. Donna Authers, *A Sacred Walk: Dispelling the Fear of Death and Caring for the Dying* (Broken Arrow, OK: A & A, 2008).

10. Maggie Callanan and Patricia Kelley, *Final Gifts: Understanding the Special Awareness, Needs and Communications of the Dying* (New York: Simon and Schuster, 2012).

9. REMEMBERING

1. Bob Tedeschi, (@bobtedeschi), April 7, 2016. "As the End Nears, 'Death Doulas' Ease the Way," STAT e-newsletter, accessed December 26, 2017, www.statnews.com/2016/04/07/death-doulas-end-of-life/.

2. MedlinePlus, focus on bereavement, accessed December 25, 2017, https://medlineplus.gov/bereavement.html/.

3. Chris Thompson writes of these events in his "Church Visits" blog, accessed December 26, 2017, https://www.churchvisits.com/2017/12/not-feeling-holiday-cheer-maybe-a-blue-christmas-or-longest-night-service-is-for-you/.

4. Stephanie Buck, "How 1 Billion People Are Coping with Death and Facebook," February 13, 2013, accessed December 17, 2017, http://mashable.com/2013/02/13/facebook-after-death/#53pN2bHdI8qI/.

5. Candi Cann, *Virtual Afterlives: Grieving the Dead in the Twenty-First Century* (Lexington: University Press of Kentucky, 2015).

6. Kate Poss, "The Final Act: Lucinda Herring Helps Families Care for Their Dead," *Whidbey Life Magazine*, April 19, 2017.

7. Find more ideas for home funerals and doulas by googling these keywords: "a sacred passing," "final passages," "crossings," "home funerals." Information can also be found through the National Home Funeral Alliance.

8. See Michael Hebb's TedMed 2017 talk at http://www.tedmed.com/talks/show?id64618, and his website accessed December 17, 2017, www.deathoverdinner.org/.

9. A touching few moments in a Garth Brooks concert as he sang "The Dance" to a cancer patient: accessed December 17, 2017, https://www.youtube.com/watch?v=veCRhOCwNEs/.

10. Maxine Harris, *The Loss that Is Forever: The Lifelong Impact of the Early Death of a Mother or Father* (New York: Plume Books, 1996).

11. Christy Whitney, *Videos for Grieving Children*, accessed December 17, 2017, http://listen2kids.net/dvd-illness-grief.html.

12. *Sesame Street* videos: accessed December 17, 2017, https://grievingtogether.ca/grief-videos-kids-3/.

13. Dougy Center, the National Center for Grieving Children and Families, focusing on grief in children: accessed December 17, 2017, https://www.dougy.org/.

10. MIXED FEELINGS ABOUT END-OF-LIFE CARE

1. National Hospital and Palliative Care Organization, *Facts and Figures, Hospice in America*, March 1, 2017, p. 5, accessed December 13, 2017, www.nhpco.org/sites/default/files/public/Statistics_Research/2016_Faces_Figures.pdf/.

2. Angela Morrow, "The Common Myths about Hospice," accessed December 18, 2017, https://www.verywell.com/hospice-myths-1132617/.

3. POLST (physician orders for sustaining life) is called by different names in different locations; it's easy to find the form for your location at this website, accessed December 23, 2017, http://polst.org/.

4. Atul Gawande, MD, *Being Mortal: Medicine and What Matters in the End* (New York: Picador 2014).

5. Ibid., 1.

6. Ibid., 8.

7. Ibid., 229.

8. Clear Conversations: https://khn.org/news/terrifying-brush-with-death-drives-doctor-to-fight-for-patients/ and https://www.compassionandchoices.org/research/doc2doc-program/, accessed March 13, 2018.

9. Kathleen Mitchell, Alan, Roth, Gina Basello, and Jeffrey Ring. "A Culturally Responsive Approach to Advance Care Planning: A New Communication Framework Tool to Reduce Racial Disparities in End-of-Life Care (TH358)," *Journal of Pain and Symptom Management* 5, no. 51 (February 2016): 339–40.

10. *National Journal* poll of 500 physicians, reported in "Living Well at the End of Life: A National Conversation," accessed December 12, 2017, http://syndication.nationaljournal.com/communications/NationalJournalRegenceToplines.pdf/.

11. Ken Murray, "How Doctors Choose to Die," *The Guardian*, February 8, 2012, accessed December 14, 2017, http://www.theguardian.com/society/2012/feb/08/how-doctors-choose-die/.

12. Dana Lustbader et al., "The Impact of a Home-Based Palliative Care Program in an Accountable Care Organization," *Journal of Palliative Medicine* 10, no. 10 (2016); Amy S. Kelley, "Hospice Enrollment Saves Money for Medicare and Improves Care Quality Across a Number of Different Lengths-of-Stay," *Health Affairs* 32, no. 3 (March 2013): 552–61.

13. National Hospice and Palliative Care Organizations Press Release, August 19, 2010, accessed December 18, 2017, https://www.nhpco.org/press-room/research-shows-patients-may-live-longer-hospice-and-palliative-care/.

11. MAKING GOOD END-OF-LIFE DECISIONS

1. America's Essential Hospitals, "History of Public Hospitals in the United States," accessed December 17, 2017, https://essentialhospitals.org/about-americas-essential-hospitals/history-of-public-hospitals-in-the-united-states/.

2. Patients need to ask their physician for details about their illness and their options for care so they can make informed decisions about treatment and "how they want to spend their remaining time," says Dr. Rab Razzale, director of outpatient palliative medicine at Johns Hopkins Medicine in Baltimore.

3. Washington State Medical Society, https://wsma.org/.

4. Angelo Volandes, *The Conversation: A Revolutionary Plan for End-of-Life Care* (New York: Bloomsbury, 2015).

5. Ellen Goodman, co-founder and director of "The Conversation Project," accessed December 17, 2017, https://theconversationproject.org/.

6. Ibid.

7. Questions and Concerns, instead of Questions and Answers, is used by Ron Jolliffe, professor of film and literature, Walla Walla University, College Place, Washington.

8. "The Conversation Project."

9. Death Over Dinner, accessed December 17, 2017, http://deathoverdinner.org/; TedTalk with Michael Heeb, entrepreneur and activist describing the beginning of this activity, accessed December 17, 2017, http://www.tedmed.com/talks/show?id_64618/.

10. Caring Community, http://www.caringcommunity.org/helpful-resources/models-research/caring-conversations/.

11. End of Life, Washington, https://endoflifewa.org/. The instructions and explanations are excellent. These documents may vary in different states. You can use these documents and have them notarized; it is recommended that you consult with an attorney.

12. REFLECTIONS

1. Elizabeth Kubler-Ross, *On Death and Dying* (New York: Macmillan, 1969). Wisdom about what the dying have to teach doctors, nurses, clergy, and their own families.

2. George Eliot, *Middlemarch* (1871; Boston, MA: Charles E. Lauriat Co., 1908), chap. 72.

APPENDIX A

1. +Widgit Health, accessed December 22, 2017, https://www.widgit-health.com/products/index.htm, and Wong-Baker FAES Scale, accessed December 22, 2017, http://www.wongbakerfaces.org/.

2. Some of these safety ideas are adapted from Tena Alonzo, director of education and research, Beatitudes Campus, a retirement community in Phoenix, Arizona, cited in "The Sense of an Ending" by Rebecca Mead, *The New Yorker*, May 20, 2013.

3. Ibid.

Index

Also see "Appendix D: Glossary, Terms, and Abbreviations"

AARP. *See* American Association of Retired Persons

acceptance. *See* grief

ACP, advance care planning. *See* advanced directives

ACS. *See* American Cancer Society

acquired immunodeficiency syndrome (AIDS), 75, 82, 83, 84, 85, 106, 151, 159n4, 159n6. *See also* human immunodeficiency virus (HIV)

activities of daily living (ADL), 139

addiction vs. dependency, 12

ADL. *See* activities of daily living

adult care homes. *See* facilities

adult day care, 55, 139

advance care planning (ACP). *See* advance directives

advance directives, xi, 115, 119, 123, 143; Advance Care Planning, 139; DNI/Do Not Intubate, 141; DNR/Do Not Resuscitate, xi, 89, 114, 141; health care proxy, 139; MOLST/POLST. See Medical Orders for Life-sustaining Treatment/Physician Orders for Life-sustaining treatment, 119, 139, 145, 159n4, 161n3; Trust, 139; Will, 139

Advocate. *See also* ombudsman, xii, 50, 53, 55, 114, 123, 143, 144, 158n6

after death care: celebration of life, 140, 142; burial, xii, 105, 142, 143, 148, 151; cremation, 140, 141; embalming, 140, 142, 148; funeral service, 17, 108, 140; green burial, xii, 105, 142, 143, 148, 151; graveside service, 26; home funeral, xii, 103, 140, 148, 160n7; memorial, xii, 5, 35, 63, 74, 103, 104, 105, 106, 107, 108, 140, 144, 151

AIDS. *See* acquired immunodeficiency syndrome

ADL. *See* activities of daily living

Allen, Woody, 97, 98, 160n8

ALS. *See* amyotrophic lateral sclerosis/ Lou Gehrig's Disease

Alternative Medicine. *See* Complementary and Alternative Medicine (CAM)

American Association of Retired Persons (AARP), 35, 46, 111, 139

American Cancer Society (ACS), ix, 34, 75, 76, 78, 110, 111, 126, 139, 169

amyotrophic lateral sclerosis (ALS)/Lou Gehrig's Disease, 29, 140, 148

ANH. *See* artificial nutrition and hydration

Alzheimer's Disease, 33, 141, 143, 157n19

ambiguous loss. *See* grief

anger, 67

anomic aphasia, 20

anorexia. *See* symptoms

anxiety. *See* symptoms

apnea/difficulty breathing. *See* symptoms

About the Author

SOCIAL WORKER, SOCIOLOGIST, TRAVELER, WRITER, BLOGGER

Karen J. Clayton is a social worker and a sociologist. She has worked in adoptions, at a residential center for adolescents, in county and private hospitals, at a hospice, and as the director of patient services for a regional office of the American Cancer Society.

Her undergraduate work was in social services and she was awarded a social work license and earned a master's degree in sociology through the University of Texas at Arlington, where she focused on cultural diversity, social problems, and belief systems. She teaches sociology and cross-cultural communication at the university level. Clayton helped initiate two community help lines and a multidisciplinary perinatal loss team in a hospital system in Texas.

She, her husband (a professor and researcher), and their adolescent daughter and son lived for three years in the Republic of the Philippines, enjoying an interesting "slice in time" under martial law during the Marcos regime. Their focus there was education; much of their time was spent being challenged by, and learning to love, the culture of Southeast Asia.

Clayton and her husband are completing a book about their adventures in Republic of the Philippines titled *The Gentle Clash of Cultures: A Lovers' Quarrel*. Chapters from *Demystifying Hospice* won second place in the 2015 Ink and Insights Nonfiction Writing Contest under the title *Tell Me Your Story*. Museums and art are special interests, and she volunteered as education curator for the Stahl Center Museum of Culture in La Sierra University. Friends and family, reading, writing, and traveling are her special joys. She and her husband live on Whidbey Island, Washington. They have two adult children living in California and Australia.

Clayton writes a travel blog titled "Cultural Adventures," sharing experiences, photographs, and insights from Australia, Canada, Belgium, Dubai, Egypt, Honduras, Hong Kong, France, Germany, Great Britain, Hawaii, India, Israel, Italy, Lichtenstein, Mexico, New Zealand, The Republic of the Philippines, Switzerland, Singapore, Tahiti, and Thailand. Travel bucket list: Ireland, Scotland, Portugal, and Spain, available at https://karenjclayton. wordpress.com/.